ANTI
INFLAMMATORY
DIET

The Smart Diet for Beginners.

14-Days No-Stress Meal Plan with Simple and Delicious Recipes.

It Helps You Heal the Immune System, Prevent Diseases, and Lose Weight Easily.

"There are only two days in the year that nothing can be done. One is called yesterday and the other is called tomorrow, so today is the right day to love, believe, do, and mostly, live."

(Dalai Lama)

Mely Johnson

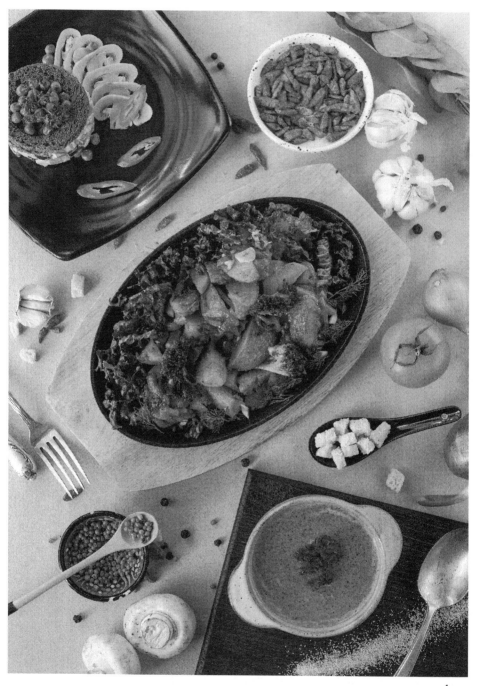

4

author is not engaging in the rendering of legal, financial, medical or professional advice. The content within this book has been derived from various sources. Please consult a licensed professional before attempting any techniques outlined in this book. By reading this document, the reader agrees that under no circumstances is the author responsible for any losses, direct or indirect, which are incurred as a result of the use of information contained within this document, including, but not limited to, — errors, omissions, or inaccuracies

TABLE OF CONTENTS

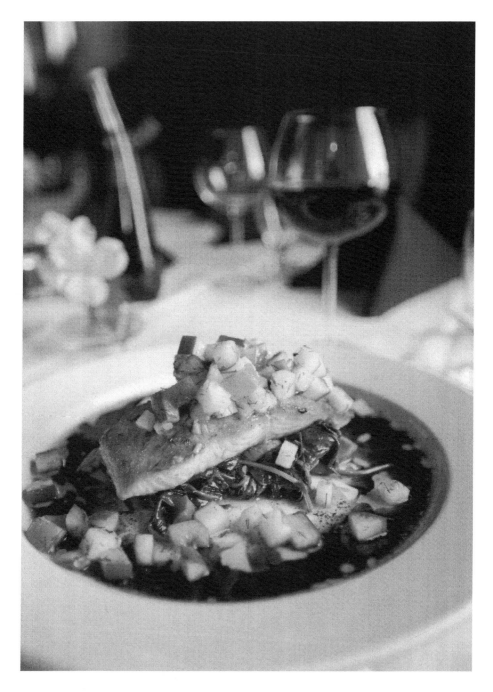

Introduction

The choices of food that you make daily affect your health today and in the future. One of the best ways of leading a healthy lifestyle is through good nutrition. It is central to maintaining a healthy Body Mass Index (BMI) and promoting your overall health.

One of the most used and yet most misunderstood health terms in everyday conversation is inflammation. You'll hear people saying that they have been ordered by a health practitioner to take on a particular diet to reduce inflammation, but they don't understand what it really means. Understanding inflammations is core to leading a healthier life. Inflammation is linked to acute and chronic health concerns, so learning what you need to do and what you need in your everyday diet will reduce the chances of inflammation. You don't have to wait until you get to chronic inflammation to watch your diet. It is good to avoid it at all costs.

This book is the ultimate guide to living an inflammation-free life and achieving higher health standards. The topics herein include:

- What inflammation is
- Foods and drinks that reduce inflammation and those that cause inflammation
- Frequently asked questions about inflammation
- Tips to reduce inflammation

Most importantly, I will provide simple and quick-fix recipes that will help you avoid inflammation.

Research shows that people across the world have become more proactive in health matters than how they were some time ago. While conventional healthcare has historically been practiced as a response to illness, there is an increasing need to shift awareness in behavior to prevent disease, rather than seek healthcare attention when it's there.

People want to maintain a healthy and youthful look and keep a wide distance from rising health concerns around the world. It is paramount to be more aware about the foods you consume since these choices are linked to most health concerns today. However, you may not be getting this from the grocery store where you purchase food. Also, depending on your schedule, you may not have the energy or time to make those complicated meals that take longer to prepare. So, is there a solution?

This guide has got you covered. It will not only show you the foods that you should eat to achieve an anti-inflammatory diet, it also shows you simple combinations of these food stuffs. Within these pages are quick fix recipes that anyone can do at home and each recipe is easy to follow. The rest of the book will describe what inflammation is all about. It will discuss the health risks associated with inflammatory foods and sources, what an anti-inflammatory diet looks like. Learn all about the foods you can eat within an anti-inflammatory diet and consider trying all the anti-inflammatory recipes we share.

Clearly, if you wish to lead a rewarding lifestyle, you must make conscious decisions on most nutrition issues. While diet fads are easy to forego over time, with the anti-inflammatory lifestyle you will try basic foods for their natural good taste and find that they are actually easy to prepare. This is the diet you will stick with.

There are a number of books, magazines, blogs, and websites that you can rely on to gather knowledge about diet plans and weight loss. But don't you think it gets confusing when there is too much information? Often people assume that dieting is all about restricting their chance to enjoy delicious food, but it is not! Dieting is way different than many people assume. It is not about limiting your chance to savor good food. Instead, it will help you stay on track while enjoying delicious food.

The major problem with dieting is that dieters aren't aware of the diet plan that they must select. You have so many options to pick from, but when you are selecting a diet, you must make sure that you are making the right choice. How can you know that you have made the right choice? If your diet plan doesn't suffocate you, it means you have picked the right one. So, it is important to find a diet that helps you become healthy without sacrificing delicious food.

The Anti-inflammatory diet is the solution to all your problems if you want to stay healthy while enjoying good food. This is not a typical diet. Instead, you can consider this as a way of living. When you follow the Anti-inflammatory diet, you will think of it as a life changing process; it is a way of living. You are not only motivated to eat healthily, but also to follow healthy habits that will impact your overall well-being. If you compare this diet to other diets, you will understand the difference, and you will realize that the Anti-inflammatory diet is more natural than any of the diets that you have come across before.

Even if you are a busy person, you can still follow the Anti-inflammatory diet. You'll be able to prepare the dish es in 20 minutes, therefore it will not take away time from your busy schedule. There are different ways to achieve weight loss and vitality, but the way the Anti-inflammatory diet helps you to achieve weight loss is simple and easy. Also, you don't have to worry about whether or not it is okay to follow this type of diet, because this is one of the oldest and most recognized diet programs.

The recipes included in this book will mesmerize you because they don't leave out all the best tastes and flavors. Even if you are dieting, you will still get the chance to enjoy delicious recipes prepared in a short time. Not only you, but everyone at the table will be pleased with the foods they will be served. You don't have to think that as a beginner, you will need a lot of time to understand this diet. You don't have to exert any additional effort to understand this diet because I'll explain everything to you in detail. All the essential information about the Anti-inflammatory diet can be learned and understood from this eBook. Plus, it is better to start with the 14-days meal plan, so I'll help you with that too and make things easier for you.

It takes only takes a few weeks to make anything a habit, it will be easy to build a healthy future. You will find recipes for breakfast, lunch, dinner, smoothies and even dessert recipes.

The following chapters will discuss how to improve your daily life, heal your immune system, lose weight and even prevent degenerative diseases. Inflammation can throw you into a cycle that is difficult to get out of causing pain in your muscles and joints leaving you less active. Living a more sedentary lifestyle will cause weight gain which will then put more pressure on your joints and cause more inflammation.

But, you can control the inflammation by just changing your way of eating you can reduce the inflammation causing fatigue, and many autoimmune diseases. You will find you no longer need pain medication daily and you don't have to starve yourself to get there!

Flip to the next page and start reading how to lead an Anti-inflammatory lifestyle!

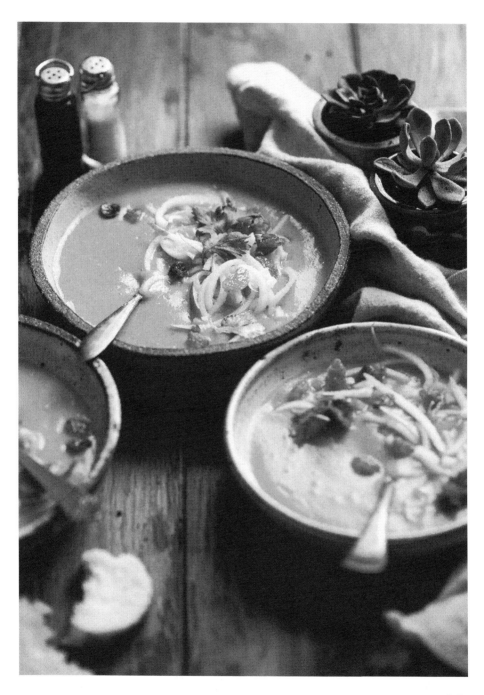

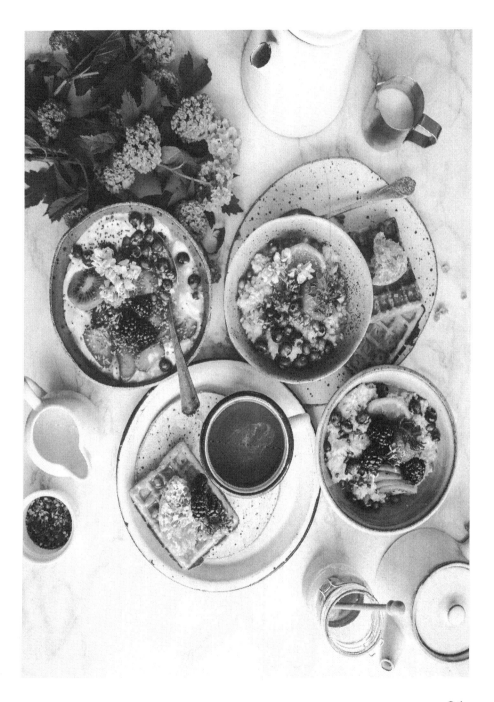

Chapter 1: What is Inflammation and What Causes it?

Inflammation is the immune system's response to injury or infection in the body. It is the process through which your white blood cells produce the means of protecting our bodies from infection by viruses and bacteria. Also, it can be referred to as a signal that the body sends to its immune system to repair damage. It is a core function of the immune system, without which wounds and infections would always be noxious.

Although it is an important part of the immune system, inflammation that occurs without an injury or persists after an injury is not a normal happening and can lead to the development of autoimmune conditions. Scientists refer to autoimmune conditions as those which arise from an abnormal response of the immune system to a body part without an issue. Whilst the immune system is created to automatically sense invaders and differentiate them from the good cells of the body, an autoimmune response mistakes your body parts for foreign elements and proceeds to attack them. These sudden attacks on the body can lead to severe health conditions such as stroke, arthritis, and heart disease.

Inflammation occurs in two modes, acute and chronic.

Acute Inflammation

Acute inflammation is a response of the immune system whereby inflammation occurs from an injury. This might be a situation where you get a cut or suffer a strained joint; inflammation occurs and lasts for a short while, fading away as the injury heals.

The most common symptoms of this mode of inflammation include swelling, a general rise of body temperature, fatigue, and loss of appetite, stiffness of muscles, pain, redness and swelling in the area of concern. The process of healing occurs through the production of cytokines, also known as emergency signals of the body. Cytokines send the body a message that the infected tissue needs white blood cells for healing. Dilation of the blood vessels near the spot occurs to allow more blood flow and more white blood cells. This process is what triggers your experience of pain, swelling, and fever, but those symptoms will gradually subside.

Chronic Inflammation

Contrary to acute inflammation, chronic inflammation has a long-lasting impact on your body. Also, instead of affecting a single part of your body as in acute mode, a chronic mode of inflammation has the potential of affecting your entire body. It occurs gradually in a steady manner and it can be judged by the rise of immune system indicators in the blood tissue. Chronic inflammation is highly likely to lead to the development of diseases. It is caused by a perceived threat in the body which prompts the immune system to respond. When white blood cells swarm the tissue without a normal function to carry out, they begin to attack healthy organs. The worst fact about chronic inflammation is that its manifestation is difficult to spot. This is a common characteristic of other chronic health conditions that develop silently, including cancer and diabetes.

The good news is that there are clinical tests that can be performed to uncover the presence of this ailment within the body. In healthcare facilities, medics mostly rely on observing the body and inquiring whether you have ever experienced any strain or discomfort in your joints. Also, medics may perform x-rays and conduct blood tests to affirm their physical and patient-doctor interview diagnosis.

Cases of acute inflammation are often easily treated with over the counter medications. Commonly used NSAID drugs and pain relievers like, naproxen, ibuprofen, and aspirin are considered safe and effective against short term inflammation. These drugs work by blocking the enzyme cyclooxygenase, which produces the prostaglandins, this reduces the pain making it more bearable. If the over-the-counter medications do not ease the discomfort, there are prescriptions that may work as well as cortisone and steroids such as prednisone that are known to reduce inflammation. Unfortunately, there are no medications specifically for treating chronic inflammation.

While there are many options to treat inflammation

NSAIDs when used often over months or years to raise the risk of stroke or heart attack as well as stomach and side effects such as ulcers and bleeding. Cortisone can cause weight gain, osteoporosis, diabetes and muscle weakness. Prednisone is prescribed to treat a wide array of symptoms and diseases but it can also suppress the immune system causing an increased risk of infection. With long term use it may also increase the risk of osteoporosis, thinning skin, fluid retention and weight gain caused by increased hunger.

Medications may act quickly and help reduce the pain for a few hours, but they may also take many daily tasks. When inflammation becomes chronic and is affecting your daily life, it 's time to begin looking for a long term solution to the inflammation. What and when when you eat ...

Researcher are still trying to understand the specifics of inflammation and what the effects are on the body but what is known is inflammatory foods are linked to a higher risk of long term and difficult to manage diseases like type 2 diabetes and heart disease.

Eating anti-inflammatory foods will calm your overactive immune system. By changing your way of eating you will not only reduce your symptoms of inflammation but you may even be able to reverse the progress of conditions you already have including: inflammatory bowel and Crohn's disease, depression, anxiety, autoimmune diseases such as lupus, psoriasis and types of arthritis, cardiovascular diseases, metabolic disorders such as diabetes, high cholesterol, asthma and even skin conditions such as eczema.

While larger scale studies are still needed, chronic inflammation has been linked to many major diseases that effect a large portion of society. Heart disease, arthritis, diabetes, Alzheimer's depression and even cancers have been linked to inflammation. In experimental studies, it was found that there are many foods that have anti-inflammatory effects. These studies have also been able to pin point many of the foods and beverages that can cause inflammation to flare up.

By choosing the right foods to eat, you can lessen the inflammation in your body, slow down or even cause current ailments to regress.

It is not surprising that the majority of foods found to cause inflammation are the foods that we have always been told are "unhealthy." We already know that eating too many unhealthy foods can cause us to gain weight, and additional weight can increase our risk of inflammation but even when obesity was taken into account, there was still an undeniable link between foods and inflammation.

A New Way of Life, A New You

You have the power to take control of your health. The Anti-Inflammatory Diet works to remove toxins and chemicals from the body that come from the average diet. While it will not work within an hour or two like pain medication will, it will reduce your chronic inflammation, increase your energy and doesn't come with all of the side effects.

When living with chronic inflammation are you really living? When fighting off chronic inflammation you endure many symptoms that can change the way you live your life. You may find yourself going out less often due to the pain or fatigue. You see the world passing you by and may miss out on time that could have been spent with friends or grandchildren. As muscles and joints become stiff from swelling you may move around less often even in your own home. This often causes weight gain which will only exacerbate the pain and inflammation. By consuming anti-inflammatory foods, you can reduce your pain and swelling within a matter of days. Once your inflammation is reduced, you will be up and moving around again in no time and be able to spend time playing with grandkids or going for a walk. You will feel the increase in your energy and know you were able to make those changes to your life by just eating healthy foods and knowing which foods to avoid.

It may seem difficult to give up so many of your favorite foods or to stick to a limited diet, but the benefits outweigh the losses. By letting go of the foods that cause inflammation you will truly be able to take control of your life and your health. You will find that if you are strict and only eat anti-inflammatory foods your taste buds will change and so will your cravings. Soon you will not miss those sugary desserts and you will find new favorites. Once you see and feel the difference as the inflammation subsides you won't look back.

Inflammation can affect you in many different ways. You may not have even realized you were not feeling your best. It may just be your normal and you didn't even know you could feel stronger or faster. You may have assumed it was natural due to aging or lack of sleep.   You will find that once you begin the Anti-Inflammatory Diet your fatigue will subside and you will be able to sleep more soundly at night.

But for lasting health, you have to go into this not thinking of it as a diet, but truly as a new way of eating, a new way of life. While inflammation can be reduced by eating the correct foods, it can just as quickly come back if you fall back into your old eating habits. You have to be ready for this change. If you're sick of feeling sick and sore everyday, you are the only one that can change that.

There currently are no long term medications to reduce chronic inflammation. You may be prescribed medications that treat some of the symptoms of inflammation, but many of those medications have side effects and can be hard on your liver and kidneys. These side effects may become so difficult to live with that you are now prescribed additional medications to treat the side effects of the first medication. It becomes a constant battle trying to get in front of it and the cost of medications and doctor's visits only makes it more frustrating and causes additional stress in your life.

Make the decision to change your life for the better, eat healthy anti-inflammatory foods, even more importantly, STOP EATING INFLAMMATORY FOODS and you will see less need for those doctor visits and medication.

Chapter 2: How Does Inflammation Effect Your Everyday Life?

Health Problems Caused by Inflammatory Foods

There are various situations and conditions that contribute to inflammation. These conditions exert physiological stress on the body, lead to high levels of sugar, and inhibit lipid digestion.

Conditions that contribute to inflammation include:

Foods we consume: Diet is by far the greatest contributor to inflammation and there are many contributing foods that we might consume. Certainly, sugary foods will increase the chances of inflammation in our blood vessels. The process through which foods cause inflammation begins in the jejunum, as our food is digested. The more foods we have within the intestines that the body views as invading rivals, the more toxins that enter our bloodstream. When your body senses foreign substances in the digestive system, it sends a message to the protective system of the body and there is an attack, a battle. As a protective measure, the system releases its counter attacking cells such as lymphocytes. The entire body strives to block these invaders from entering into every cell and this leads to inflammation in the overall bloodstream. Therefore, eating unhealthily is a great contributor to inflammation and severe infections.

Failure to eliminate whatever is causing acute inflammation: Further, inflammation in your bloodstream prevents sufficient sugar from getting into the brain cells. Since brain cells need sugar to function, you end up needing more glucose and feeding into more sugary foodstuffs to get the glucose. The ultimate result of this is chronic inflammation.

Eating habits: Poor eating habits like hasty eating stresses the body and at times like this the body is unable to absorb nutrients needed to keep you healthy.

Stress: A strong link exists between stress and anxiety and instances and aggravation of inflammation yet the crucial central nervous system is one of the most overlooked elements in the body's inflammatory process.

It is good to understand that CNS triggers the immune process to respond to tissue injury or infection.

Stress and anxiety activate the inflammatory pathway and can also develop the body's urge to consume those inflammatory foods even when we are not hungry. Stress feeding, with calorie-filled and nutrient-poor foods furthers the cycle and endorses the condition of being overweight, which is known to cause inflammation.

Socio-economic environment: the environment that you live in may influence your lifestyle, which will in turn influence your immune system. You community may make you believe that you have to eat something, even though it feels like your body does not work well with it. Income will impact your ability to sustain all of your needs; you may not be able to afford a costly anti-inflammatory diet. Unfortunately, you may not even know which low-cost foods are also part of the anti-inflammation diet.

Scientists argue that when the inflammatory cells stay for long in the blood, they lead to a condition known as plague. The plague is perceived by the immune system as a foreign invader in the body and as such, your system strives to prevent the plague within the blood vessels from getting inside arteries. Over time, the plague may become wobbly and rupture, forming a lump that blocks sufficient blood flow throughout the body. Consequently, this leads to the condition of stroke or heart attack, otherwise known as cardiovascular disease (CVD) and among the highest cause of mortality in the developed nations.

Cancer

Usually, chronic inflammation that lasts and persists within the body leads to damage of the Deoxyribonucleic acid (DNA), and which ultimately causes tumor development.

Type 2 Diabetes

Being unable to produce sufficient insulin, a chemical

responsible for maintaining sustainable levels of blood sugar, is a characteristic inherent in Diabetes victims. Scientists have found out that people whose blood sugar is unregulated have higher inflammation levels than people without. The implication of this is that low-grade inflammation alters the action of insulin in the body, and hence can cause Diabetes 2.

Arthritis

Arthritis is a major inflammation related condition. Arthritis is described as an inflammation of the joints. While inflammation is connected to rheumatoid arthritis and gouty arthritis, some types of arthritis like osteoarthritis are not caused by inflammation.

Treatment for Chronic Inflammation

As previously mentioned, inflammation is part of the healing process, in the case of infected tissues. However, sometimes reducing inflammation is also helpful. There are anti-inflammatory drugs, herbs, and supplements on the market today.

Although to date, no drug has been found whose direct

function is to cure chronic inflammation, there are over the counter medicines which can treat and help manage the symptoms of acute or chronic inflammation. These medicines include aspirin and ibuprofen which are classed within the category of non-fat insoluble drugs. They work by destroying the substances that cause inflammation and can provide relief from the pain and fever associated with inflammation. However, when taken over a long period of time, these drugs can lead to the development of other infections which manifest as severe side effects, so these drugs should be avoided as a long-term solution.

For cases of chronic inflammation, medicines which include ingredients like prednisone and cortisone are prescribed to stop inflammation. They contain the steroid hormone which combats inflammation. The consumption of these drugs come with the potential for negative side effects like fluid retention and weight gain. Other drugs may come in the form of salves, often used to treat inflammation in the lungs, bowels, eyes, and skin.

Devil's claw is a recognized dietary supplement that acts as an effective suppressor of severe inflammation, although the evidence available today of their usage is limited. Besides this, herbs such as Hyssop oils, Turmeric, Ginger and Cannabis are known to inhibit the development of inflammatory reactions within the body system. They have been used in the concept of disease treatment and prevention long into the history of our human civilization and they have been effective in relieving arthritis pains and soreness in the lungs, among other illnesses. Apart from Cannabis, herbs are easily available in most areas. In the case of the Cannabis herb, the legislation around its possession and use varies from place to place.

Overall, anti-inflammatory diets and positive changes in lifestyle are among the most efficient and fulfilling treatments for inflammation. Not only does a diet that consists of anti-inflammatory foods suppress our levels of inflammation, this diet also helps to prevent inflammation. Not surprisingly, anti-inflammatory diets have become a common cure for chronic inflammation.

Chapter 3: Benefits of the Anti-Inflammatory Diet

A study conducted by Estruch in 2010 and published by the Cambridge University Press linked adherence to the typical Mediterranean diet, also known as Med-Diet, to lower cardiovascular (CVD) risks. Estruch explored the use of Med-Diet on the cellular biomarkers and serum associated with atherosclerosis (plague). Using nuts and virgin olive oils on a sample of 722 subjects presenting a high risk of CVD, it was identified that subjects following the Med-Diet produced more favorable results than those experienced by subjects on a simple low-fat diet. Med-Diet subjects portrayed improved blood pressure, improved digestion of lipids and improved insulin function. Results from this study endorsed the Mediterranean diet as an effective intervention for CVD.

A subsequent study was done by Lucas, Russell, and Keast, and published by Bentham Science publishers in 2011 established that the phenolic compound, oleocanthal, found in virgin olive oil is an effective intervention key to curing most conditions associated with inflammation, including heart disease, some types of cancer and diabetes. The research was based on the scientific background that virgin olive oil contains the same anti-inflammatory elements as ibuprofen, such as oleocanthal. Therefore, it verified therapeutic action and anti-inflammatory potential. The researchers endorsed its usage as a natural intervention, rather than using the drugs because they have severe side effects.

N-3 fatty acids have been found to be effective in controlling conditions such as inflammatory bowel disease, diabetes, CVD, and also septic and septicemia shock, based on a study published in the Elsevier Science Direct Journal. The subjects under study were of Japanese and Eskimo heritage and were put under a diet full of fish oil. The main focus was the N-3 fatty acids found in fish oil and their influence on inflammation. The result was that these fatty acids had an overall direct impact on Arrhythmogenesis. Based on the analysis, the fatty acid's main action is to curb the development of cytokines known to cause heart disease.

An empirical study connecting diet and body tissue was conducted with the aim of guiding dietary decisions. The study was published by the New York Academy of Sciences in 2006. The study had the major implication that increasing the consumption of omega 3 fatty acids, as well as closely managing the amount of food being eaten in each meal to reduce oxidant stress, are effective ways of suppressing conditions associated with inflammation. This study contributed to the awareness about effective diets for suppressing inflammation levels in the body and the healthy eating habits that we should adopt. It offered primary interventions in preventing the major cause of diseases today.

Another study published by the SpringerLink publisher in 2009 held that flavonoids found in the Med-Diet have the potential to act as therapeutic agents that treat inflammatory diseases. Some of the core actions of flavonoids include anti-oxidation and toning down the development of pro-inflammatory agents. The study established that flavonoids attenuate inflammatory responses in our bodies. This research indicates that foodstuffs such as tea, berries, and legumes containing flavonoids are effective anti-inflammatory foods.

Chapter 4: Disease Prevention with the Anti-Inflammatory Diet

Health practitioners recommend food choices consistent with the Mediterranean diet, full of vegetables and fresh fruits, which science has shown beyond a doubt helps to protect the body against the damages of inflammation. Many recipe ingredients typical of Mediterranean cuisine then are among the food choices that make up the anti-inflammatory diet.

A large part of the anti-inflammatory diet is that people stay away from foods that encourage inflammation. Prevention is the best course of action, so understanding how inflammatory foods infiltrate our bloodstream and how this reaches a chronic or serious level is so important.

As observed above, prolonged low-grade inflammation, popularly termed chronic inflammation, occurs over a long period of time. Therefore, experts suggest that our dietary food choices can actually curb critical inflammatory trails. Some understanding of how individual nutrients impact on the same targets that inflammatory is essential here. Ideally, a diet should be made up of the appropriate number of calories, and contains lots of soluble fiber, monounsaturated fatty acids, and polyphenols. A high omega 3 - omega 6 ratio and few refined carbohydrates is good for inflammation purposes. This is a diet that focuses on nutrient-rich foods instead of sugary refined food.

A Mediterranean diet pattern, which as the name suggests, is based on the feeding habits found in the Mediterranean region. Therefore, it's most suitable for anti-inflammation. Its recipes contain vegetables, fish, fruits, healthy fats, and whole grains. Strong observance of this diet has shown tremendous chances of health improvement. Combined with good levels of physical activity, the Mediterranean diet is one of the healthiest regimens, used not only for anti-inflammation but for maintaining an overall good health condition.

The rationale behind the dietary and lifestyle interventions to conditions of anti-inflammation is one that has been used in various health and fitness concepts. People must be ready to make conscious decisions regarding everything they do that has an impact on their health. An important aspect of an anti-inflammatory diet is it includes antioxidants which reduce the risk of inflammatory comebacks of the body and thereby, the development of associated health concerns already discussed.

The full benefits of committing to anti-inflammatory nutrition cannot be understated. As you reduce the consumption of substances that lead to or intensify inflammation, you free yourself from its various implications. It has already been established that most of the inflammatory bacteria in our bodies don't come from anything weirder than the foods you consume daily. Most of the foods that cause inflammation have a relatively low nutritional value. Therefore, replacing these foods is great for your body and makes for a more rewarding life.

An anti-inflammatory diet is credited by naturopaths, dietitians, and doctors as a suitable therapy for numerous conditions a person may experience due to chronic inflammation, including Lupus, heart disease, metabolic syndrome, obesity, diabetes, and inflammatory bowel disease. Furthermore, it can help in dealing with Colitis, Crohn's Disease, Eosinophilic Esophagitis, Asthma, Psoriasis, and Rheumatoid Arthritis.

We know that diet plays a pivotal role in addressing the issue of inflammation. We also know a suitable anti-inflammatory diet provides a good balance of fats, carbs, and protein in each meal along with water, fiber, minerals, and vitamins. Some of the anti-inflammatory foods we look at in this book include cherries, berries, tomatoes, green leafy vegetables, and whole grains, among others. Together, these provide protective compounds such as antioxidants.

The Mediterranean diet is also called the heart-healthy diet; however, you can call it whatever you'd like. If you follow this diet, you don't have to give up on delicious living because it doesn't deprive you from eating your favorite delicious foods. When you check out the 14-Days meal plan outlined in this book, you will realize that it's in fact an enjoyable diet. The Mediterranean diet has been considered the best by many medical professionals. The University of Barcelona conducted a study in 2013 that had proved that the Mediterranean diet has a positive impact on cardiovascular health.

Even though the research was done in the early stages, the results of the research were not taken into consideration. But later, many experts started investigating and helped the public be more informed about the diet. Now, it has become one of the best diets in the United States because it helps to fight against a more significant percentage of health diseases. This includes health risks such as obesity, heart attack, diabetes, cholesterol. Much more can be fought against by following the Mediterranean diet.

Essentially, the Mediterranean diet is about old eating habits, mostly followed by people in countries like Italy, Greece, France, Spain, and Northern Africa. This way of eating helps to maintain good relations with family and friends as well because it encourages dining together.

Moreover, unlike other diets, the Mediterranean diet motivates people to engage in exercise. Exercising is another essential part of the Mediterranean diet, and it can be anything from walking to work or engaging in a morning walk. Most beginners confuse a Mediterranean diet with a low fat and vegetarian diet. It is not a low-fat diet because you are encouraged to consume fat. But you must not consume trans or saturated fats that are found in processed and red meats (there is a rule for the consumption of red meat). Also, it is not a vegetarian diet, even though it is highly plant-based, because people in the Mediterranean region consume seafood and fish.

If you are following this enjoyable diet, you will be able to see its effects on your overall health and body if you remain consistent. You should enjoy each bite you take because mindful eating helps a lot in controlling weight gain. The high-fiber content food will keep you full for an extended period of time, in which case you won't overeat. Also, you should make water your favorite drink so that you will drink it regularly and remain hydrated. Remaining hydrated is essential if you want your body to function properly. The Mediterranean diet wasn't primarily introduced for the purpose of weight loss; however, later on it was intended for that purpose.

You will come to understand that it is because of the plant-based food consumption and reduction of sugar and meat consumption which will impact your weight in a positive way. Luckily, you don't have to count calories like you do in other diets, which means there's less work for you to do. Plus, when considering the health benefits of the Mediterranean diet, both holistic and medical perspectives are met. There are a number of benefits that we'll discuss below. However, this is a logical and straightforward diet lifestyle that you can follow without much effort or difficulties.

A nutritionally balanced plate recommended by the Mediterranean diet looks colorful and flavorful. You will love the textures as well. When you read the recipes, you will not be able to resist making them because almost all the recipes are mouthwatering. Not feeling restrictive is the best part of the Mediterranean diet. However, you should first learn about the six important components of the Mediterranean diet:

1. **Vegetables:** The versatile and nutritious plant-based foods make the diet exciting and colorful. You must include vegetables in your meal in any form: steamed, grilled, raw, picked, or even roasted. You can easily add vegetables to the meal that you are enjoying, but you

must ensure that you roast or grill as to match with the meal.

2.   **Fruits:** The Mediterranean diet includes avocados, olives, figs, grapes, and more. These fruits are full of antioxidants and fiber. There are no limitations on how much fruit you can eat, but if you are specifically focused on the best time of day to eat them, it is best to eat fruits when you have sugar cravings.

3.   **Proteins:** Shellfish and fish are essential to add to your meal because of the protein they offer. There are healthy seafood options such as arctic char, salmon, oysters, mackerel, and anchovies. Not only animal proteins, but you can also consume plant proteins. Foods such as seeds, legumes, nuts, and beans contain unsaturated fats. Sometimes, you can use them as snacks as well.

4.   **Whole grains:** Whole grains are an ideal part of the Mediterranean diet because of their antioxidant, fiber, and anti-inflammatory properties. Whole grains such as oats, brown rice, quinoa, farro, amaranth, and much more are part of the Mediterranean diet.

5. **Healthy fats:** Olive oil is the most recommended type of oil in the Mediterranean diet. This should be used for baking, cooking, dressing, and more. Along with oil, you can consider safflower, peanut, and canola oil as per the recommendation of the American Heart Association.

6. **Red wine:** A moderate consumption of red wine is recommended as it is good for cholesterol and has many de-stressing qualities. It can also add more flavor to your meal.

History and Overview of the Mediterranean Diet

Now that you have an understanding of what the Mediterranean diet is, it is time to learn the history behind it. Just from the term "Mediterranean," you can already guess that this diet comes from the Mediterranean region and involves coastal cuisine. Among all the other cultural achievements in the Mediterranean region, one of the best achievements that became popular is the Mediterranean diet. Mediterranean countries such as Israel, Lebanon, Syria, Palestine, and more, were the first ones to cultivate cereal and legumes agriculture. Over time, the Romans and Greeks joined them to produce the basic foods that can be found in the Mediterranean diet, including wheat, olives, and more.

The Cretans were influential in the Mediterranean region, then Phoenicians emergence happened. Even the Romans and Greeks came into power, and later, the Mediterranean region became a common place where people of different faiths, cultures, religions, languages, and customs interacted. Hence, their lifestyle and eating habits all merged from different cultures. For example, the Mediterranean diet consists of Middle Age practices from the Roman tradition. The Greek diet consists of wine, oil, and bread, so you can see how eating habits of the Mediterranean diet merges two cultures together.

According to the Roman tradition, the wealthy class was blessed with fresh fish and seafood, and therefore, because of their wealthy power, they were able to consume whatever food they wanted. The poor were offered food such as olives, salted fish, and seldom meat.

Luckily, the tradition of the Romans clashed when food importing emerged. Food importing was dealt by Germanic nomads, and so their culture became an influence on eating patterns. Yet, the Roman culture was not ready to change their style of eating. The Germanic and Christian Roman Empire formed a new culture for food. But that was not all, because the southern Mediterranean shore and region managed to develop their own culture.

With time, Muslims played a role in the diet by introducing plant-based foods that were consumed by the wealthy. Foods like citrus, sugar cane, spinach, eggplant, and more were highly priced and not affordable by the middle-class. Hence, Islamic culture had played a huge role in the transformation of Mediterranean food.

When Europeans discovered America, new diet patterns emerged, thus the introduction of a new culinary tradition and of new foods including corn, tomatoes, potatoes, chili, beans, and peppers. In fact, a tomato wasn't considered edible until then, and it was later introduced into the Mediterranean diet. Even though vegetables are centralized in the Mediterranean tradition, cereals play an important role in feeding the poor and treating hunger pangs. However, the type of cereal and the method of preparing it will differ among traditions and geographical connotation of the population of countries near the Mediterranean region.

If you clearly understand the above historical events, you will be able to see the similarities between the diets of today and the Mediterranean diet. The lifestyle of people, who live in the Mediterranean regions, and their history, play a massive role in the Mediterranean diet. This dieting model focuses on the social, historical, environmental, and cultural elements; therefore, it is appreciated universally.

Ultimately, the Mediterranean diet is a food model that helps to develop healthy eating habits to ensure a healthy lifestyle. Even though there are simple cuisines in the Mediterranean diet, you will rarely need to sacrifice the taste of the food, which is ultimately the best part about the diet. The health of individuals will be positively impacted when they follow the Mediterranean diet.

Health Benefits of the Mediterranean Diet

Once you have understood the definition, history, and overview of the diet, you should learn about the health benefits this diet has to offer. Below, I've outlined various information on the benefits related to heart health, weight loss, brain health, bones, diabetes, blood sugar, cancer, depression, anxiety, menopause, gut, longevity, etc. Now, let's discuss some of the benefits in detail.

Improves Heart Health

In previous years, various studies were unable to prove the benefits of this diet on heart health, until a study published in the New England Journal of Medicine outlines its benefits. The study focused on two different Mediterranean diets. The first diet recommended 30 grams of nuts every day, which included hazelnuts, almonds, and walnuts. The second diet recommended adding four tablespoons of extra-virgin oil to different foods every day. Researchers of this study compared these two Mediterranean diets to a low-fat diet. A low-fat diet discourages oil, nuts, and meat consumption.

Three diets, including low-fat diet, were randomly tested on 7,000 participants, men and women, aged 55-80 years, from Spain, and who were at a high risk for cardiovascular disease and type 2 diabetes. The time period of the study was five years. Results were published in 2013, when suddenly it generated flaws to which the researchers had to consider reanalyzing the data. This study's primary downfall was due to randomly assigning diets to the participants. After a few more tries, it was confirmed that the Mediterranean diet lowers rates of heart disease by 30% when compared to the low-fat diet. This study proved that the Mediterranean diet defeats the once popular low-fat diet.

Heart diseases such as stroke, myocardial infarction, and more can be controlled by taking part in the Mediterranean diet. This diet shows positive results related to the risk factors linked to cardiovascular disease, including triglycerides, cholesterol, and high blood pressure. Foods such as, oils, seafood, and antioxidant-rich foods help to fight against cardiovascular diseases.

Improves Brain Health

Healthy fats are great for brain health. A study carried out by Hellenic Longitudinal Investigation of Ageing and Diet, has proven that those who take part in the Mediterranean diet face less risk for Alzheimer's. There is a direct link between Alzheimer's risk rate and fish consumption, and the risk of developing Alzheimer's disease lowers when one increases their consumption of fish.

Researchers compared the Mediterranean diet to the MIND diet, which is the Mediterranean and DASH ("DASH or Mediterranean," 2015) diets combined together. The MIND diet consists of nuts, beans, berries, leafy and regular vegetables, seafood, olive oil, whole grains, poultry, and wine; it restricts the consumption of fast foods. More than 5,000 participants were included in the study. Researchers of the study analyzed their attention, memory, and other cognitive abilities.

After thorough analysis, they compared the results of the participants who follow a normal diet and those who follow a MIND and Mediterranean diet. The results were positive in regard to their brain health, which proved that the MIND and Mediterranean diets were considered better when compared to other diets. More importantly, people who followed the Mediterranean diet showed a 35% lower rate of risks in relation to brain health. As per the study people are encouraged to follow the Mediterranean diet if they wish to improve their overall brain health.

Contributes to Weight Loss

As previously mentioned, the Mediterranean diet does not directly contribute to weight loss. It is important to know that managing your weight will help you control any sort of weight gain or loss. By following the Mediterranean diet, you will have control over your weight because the fibers which you will have an impact on your weight. You will be consuming high fiber-enriched foods, which will keep your weight under control while supporting your metabolism. It's important you replace carbohydrates with fruits, vegetables, beans, and legumes that are rich in fiber. The key to maintaining a healthy weight is to make sure you maintain healthy eating habits while following the diet. If you go off track, do not be too hard on yourself. Instead, keep your motivations clear, stay focused, and you will not derail from your goals.

You can't expect quick results if you are following the Mediterranean diet, because like with any diet, it takes time. This diet controls weight sustainably and safely. In a study published in The Lancet: Diabetes and Endocrinology, researchers illustrate differences in the weight loss differences of participants who added olive oil and nuts to their diet and those who strictly only followed a low-fat diet. The study showed that those who followed a Mediterranean diet, and who added olive oil and nuts to their foods, had higher rates of weight loss than those who actively participated in a low-fat diet.

It's important you don't look for quick methods to lose weight as they can sometimes be dangerous. The study above showed that losing weight is possible; however, adopting the right type of diet will greatly contribute to that weight loss. As we can see, a Mediterranean diet will help you lose weight faster than a low-fat diet or any other type of diet would.

Improves Bone Health

There have been several studies conducted on the benefits that a Mediterranean diet has on bone health.

Many studies have shown that there is a lower rate of osteoporosis among people who live in the Mediterranean region. Their eating habits could be one of the major reasons for this because they consume a lot of olive oil along with vegetables and fruits. Olive oil contains the required components for maturation and proliferation of cells in the bones.

In a recent study carried out by the University of East Anglia, researchers were able to prove the benefits of the Mediterranean diet on bone health. The foods included in the Mediterranean diet greatly contribute to an individual's healthy bone conditions. The study consisted of over 1,000 participants, aged between 65-79 years old. The participants were split into two groups, one group following the Mediterranean diet, and the other group not following the diet. After 12 months, participants returned with the results and the researchers noticed that the Mediterranean diet had positive effects on those who already had osteoporosis. There had been improvements in their bone health. Those who had perfectly normal bone health and did not have osteoporosis had not shown any discernible results.

Many types of studies are being carried out in regard to the benefits of the diet on bone health, and thus far, there are no downsides to following a Mediterranean diet, according to the experts. Whether you have osteoporosis or not, this diet will surely benefit you!

Fights Against Type 2 Diabetes

The Mediterranean diet consists of quinoa, buckwheat, and much more unrefined carbohydrates. Including these foods in your diet helps to keep your blood sugar levels stabilized while still having complete energy. The Mediterranean diet fights against type 2 diabetes and provides other related benefits. This diet also greatly benefits those who had cardiovascular disease or Type 2 Diabetes.

More than 400 participants, between the ages of 50-80, were studied over a period of four years to check whether they were diagnosed with type 2 diabetes. Among the participants who followed a nuts and olive oil-based diet, 52% showed lower risk in relation to Type 2 Diabetes. This result was based on food control without the involvement of any exercise.

The meta-analysis published in the American Journal of Clinical Nutrition showed that the Mediterranean diet, in comparison to low-carbohydrate, high-protein, and low-glycemic diets, had a positive impact on an individual's blood sugar levels. It also helped to reduce the risk rate of type 2 diabetes. Hence, it is clear from this study that the Mediterranean diet is one of the best ways to prevent and reduce the risk rate of type 2 diabetes.

Reduces Risk of Cancer

It is completely possible for one to reduce their risk of cancer if one follows the Mediterranean diet. Based on various studies, people with high adherence to the diet showed a 13% lower rate of cancer. Different types of cancers can be prevented by following the Mediterranean diet, including prostate, gastric, liver, breast, colorectal, neck and head, gastric, and colon cancer. Many studies have been conducted to show that the Mediterranean diet can in fact prevent cancer, even though it limits to certain types.

Reduces Symptoms of Depression and Anxiety

There is a reason as to why psychiatrists add healthy fats and vegetable-based diets to their mental health programs. Foods like eggs, spinach, and kale contain carotenoids, which aid in changing your mood into being more optimistic and also aid in boosting healthy bacteria in the gut. In one study, researchers state that depression was less common in older people when they opted to follow a Mediterranean diet. Based on their analysis, the eating habits of this diet showed positive impacts related to depression. The research analysis posted in the journal of Molecular Psychiatry, found that 33% of people are at lower risk for depression when following a Mediterranean diet.

Reduces Symptoms of Menopause

The Mediterranean diet provides positive results on muscle and bone health for women who are in menopause. Normally, menopause has a negative impact on women's bone and muscle mass.

In a study carried out by the Universidade Federal do Rio Grande do Sul, it showed that there was an improvement in muscle and bone mass when women followed the Mediterranean diet. Women in menopause who also followed the Mediterranean diet were in good shape when compared to the ones who were not on the diet plan.

Improves Gut Health

In one study, researchers showed that those who follow the Mediterranean diet tend to have good bacteria in their gut in comparison to those who follow other western diets. The highly plant-based diet helps to increase the count of good bacteria early on. Hariom Yadav, Ph.D., carried out research on the Mediterranean diet and gut health, and published his studies in the journal Frontiers in Nutrition. In one specific study, research was not carried out on humans but rather on monkeys. Around 20 monkeys were monitored by randomly limiting their access to the Mediterranean and Western diets. This study was carried out for a month, and both diets consisted of a similar amount of calories.

Fish oil, butter, olive oil, fish, egg, wheat flour, bean flour, vegetable juice, fruit puree, and sucrose were a part of the Mediterranean diet. Butter, beef tallow, eggs, sucrose, corn syrup, and lard were included in the Western diet. The samples of the fecal were tested at the end of the month to compare the results. The good bacteria formed in the gut of monkeys which were fed Western diet foods was 0.5%, while the monkeys which were fed the Mediterranean diet foods was around 7%. The study showed that the higher percentage of good bacteria contained lactobacillus and increased in the group that followed the Mediterranean diet. Lactobacillus is a prominent bacterium required for digestion and good gut health. Therefore, the Mediterranean diet is encouraged if you want to improve gut health.

Improves Life Expectancy

Let's talk about the benefits of the Mediterranean on longevity. The primary reason for longevity is good heart health. In one Harvard study, researchers showed that telomeres in your body are protected when you follow the Mediterranean diet. The length of telomeres is one's aging biomarker. Therefore, short telomeres lower life expectancy and will increase your chances of developing chronic diseases.

The research was conducted on more than 4,000 women, and stated that when an individual follows the Mediterranean diet, they will impact their telomeres positively. Even a small change concerning the diet will have a positive impact on your overall health.

Now that you have an overview of the diet, it is time to read up on some of its restrictions!

Chapter 5: Positive Mindset, Foods to Eat on an Anti-Inflammatory Diet

It is already clear that chronic inflammation largely results from lifestyle factors such as your level of physical exercise, stress and anxiety, and most of all the food we consume each day. To reduce inflammation, avoid and/or manage these causative factors and adapt daily good habits that reduce inflammation in your life.

Anti-inflammation dietary tips:

- Consume daily servings of antioxidant foods like vegetables, sweet potatoes, and nuts

- Take in lots of water, at least 6 glasses per day. If a plain glass of water is just not your thing, spice it up by adding lemon or ginger to it. Why not transform regular water into a hot tea. For a touch of anti-inflammatory properties, you could add lemon, ginger, turmeric, and a little honey

- Avoid red meat intake and substitute with lean poultry, beans, and lentils as these are healthier proteins

- Substitute vegetable oils with olive oils

- Substitute refined carbohydrates, such as white bread and rice, for whole-grain foods like oats and brown rice or bread

- Follow a vegan, keto or Med diet to minimize your carbohydrate intake

- Use seasonings, such as garlic, ginger, and turmeric instead of salt

- Increase your consumption of n-3 fatty acids such as deep-sea fish and walnuts and minimize your intake of n-6 fatty acids

Lifestyle tips:
- Avoid stress

Stress is a major threat to the health of a person. Stress leads to various ailments including headaches, sleep deprivation, and even serious illnesses like diabetes and obesity. As identified earlier, conditions such as these are connected to inflammation. Their presence in your body puts you at risk of suffering from chronic and fatal inflammatory illnesses.

There are a number of things you can do to avoid stress. There are mindfulness exercises which can help you to connect with your inner self. For a regular routine, yoga exercises can help to relax and build a positive self-image, whatever you are going through in life. It is always good to just relax and work on accessing those deeper parts of your brain, from whence you can begin to sharpen your control over your own thoughts and behaviors. Meditation is a powerful tool that has been effective for stress release. Even the most successful people meditate on a daily basis to endorse their self-awareness and enhance emotional health. You should look for a moment in every day, maybe early each morning before you start your day or right before you go to sleep, to reflect on what has been happening with you and to relax your mind.

- Adapt good daily habits

A healthy diet is more effective alongside healthy life choices, if you are keen on what you choose to eat and spend your time doing. Some of the most instrumental daily practices for health and wellbeing are taking time to engage in physical exercise and journaling. Physical exercises complement the healthy anti-inflammatory diet that you propose to integrate into your life. It helps to keep your body in shape and also helps you avoid diseases such as cardiovascular condition and diabetes.

Journaling can help you develop mindfulness, reflecting on what you have been doing right or wrong, and how you react to life's situations. Journaling can also help you to keep on track with the anti-inflammatory diet. By looking back, you can make good food decisions with consideration for how easy to prepare or delicious a meal was. When you journal, you become true to yourself and it can help you keep focused and stick to healthy habits and a healthy diet.

- Exercise intermittent fasting

Fasting intermittently is one of the most beneficial practices for overall health. It is linked to various health benefits such as the management of weight, health of the brain as well as fighting chronic conditions like cancer and diabetes. Although most people use this practice for weight loss, you can also incorporate it into your anti-inflammatory health journey. You will be provided with a 14-days meal plan, but you could choose to skip breakfast, lunch, or dinner and allow your body fast anywhere from 12-36 hours.

Chapter 6: Foods Allowed on This Diet

Anti-Inflammatory Foods

Anti-inflammatory foods to consider are those rich in antioxidants, omega 3-fatty acids, as well as culinary herbs

Foods rich in antioxidants include:

Apples

Cherries

Berries (blackberries, blueberries and raspberries)

Avocados

Dark green leafy vegetables (spinach, kale, etc.)

Broccoli

Sweet potatoes

Nuts (almonds, walnuts, hazelnuts, etc.)

Artichokes

Whole grains (brown rice, brown bread, oats)

Dark chocolate

Beans (black, red and pinto beans)

Foods rich in omega-3 fatty acids include:

Walnuts

Fortified foods (milk and eggs)

Flaxseed

Oily deep sea fish (herring, sardines, anchovies, mackerel)

Healthy oils (omega 3 oils from nuts and fish, olive oil)

Culinary herbs and spices

- Turmeric
- Garlic
- Ginger
- Rosemary
- Cayenne
- Cinnamon

Anti-Inflammatory Drinks

The value of anti-inflammatory drinks cannot be underestimated. They are great for controlling the symptoms of inflammation, such as muscle pain and fever. They are relatively easy to prepare and can be consumed at any time of the day. Furthermore, drinks are easier to digest hence they act quicker in the body than foods.

These include:

Water

It is one of the most crucial yet most overlooked drinks. Its significance in suppressing inflammation cannot be understated. Water is good for hydration as well as cleansing. It helps to flush out toxins from the body and slows down the actions of the inflammatory response. Water, especially when spiced up with lemon, ginger or turmeric is good for anti-oxidation; hence anti-inflammation. Lemon has alkalizing properties hence it boosts oxidation.

Fruit juices that boost the digestive process, including pineapple, tart and lemon juice

Apple Cider Vinegar

Apple cider vinegar is a highly effective drink for amending the immune system. It is more of a sweet, spiced drink made of apple cider vinegar, water, lemon, cayenne pepper, and honey. The advantages come from apple cider vinegar and lemon that helps speed up the digestive tract and from ginger and cayenne to soothe an inflamed stomach.

Turmeric Tea

Although it has a very particular taste, Turmeric is excellent for muscle and gut health. When making a turmeric tea you need turmeric powder, honey, lemon, cinnamon and ground ginger. Turmeric tea will reduce stiffness and pain and provide a cure for upset stomach.

Pineapple and Ginger Juice

Unlike the other drinks in this list, Pineapple ginger juice is pleasantly sweet to taste. Its components make it both tasty and effective in dealing with stomach pain. To make this, you will require spinach, ginger, apple, lemon, pineapple, cucumber, and celery stalks. Ginger and celery reduce stomach and bowel inflammation while pineapples contain bromelain which helps the body to recover. Lemon is suitable for reducing the body's acidity while the other ingredients will provide your body with vitamins C, A, K, manganese, and folate.

Berry Beet Blast Smoothie

A great smoothie for when you are battling an upset stomach, the ingredients to use in preparing this drink include turmeric, ginger, strawberries, beets, oranges, and coconut water. Besides helping that upset stomach, this berry beet blast smoothie is a reliable source of manganese, potassium, folate and vitamin C.

Golden Chai Latte

What you need is non-dairy milk such as 2 ½ cashew milk, a cup of water, 1 teaspoon ground turmeric, a pinch of nutmeg, cinnamon, and cardamom, 2 teaspoons loose leaf chai tea and 1 tablespoon maple syrup. To prepare you will need to pour water and 2 cups of cashew milk in a medium-sized pot and warm over medium heat. Add loose-leaf chai in a tea strainer and add the water/milk mixture. Add spices and boil and remove it from heat before it fully boils. Allow it to cool for 5 minutes. Stir in the maple syrup. Pour chai tea into a glass and pour the ½ cup shew milk atop, sprinkle with cinnamon and nutmeg.

Celery Juice

In preparing this, one needs a bunch of organic celery which are blended, and the juice which is squeezed fresh. You may find its taste strong. In such a situation it is advisable to use a flavor. However, you will get maximum benefits by consuming celery alone.

Inflammatory Foods to Avoid

The foods to avoid are just as important as the ones we must include, when following an anti-inflammatory diet. To maximize the benefits, you'll feel when eating foods that combat or prevent inflammation, you should try to avoid these foods as much as possible:

Soda, cookies, doughnuts, cakes, and sweets: The food items listed here do not contain the proper amount of nutrients. They are foods that are easy to overeat which could lead to high cholesterol, high blood sugar and weight gain. Each of these conditions is also related to inflammation. It is important to know that sugar makes the body to release cytokines. It is recommended that a person cut out all added sugars, including honey and agave, when consuming anti-inflammatory diet.

Fried foods such as deep fried potatoes: The fats in these foods are saturated fats, known to inhibit proper functioning of the body's protective system. Most people assume that when they cook fried foods with healthy oils such as sunflower oil, this makes it healthy. Beware though, because if your body gets too much omega-6, it creates an imbalance between omega-3s and omega-6s, leading to inflammation.

Processed meat (sausage, hotdogs): The bad thing with this form of food is that they contain such high fat levels which will lead to inflammation if you continue to consume large amounts on a daily basis.

Dairy products (ice cream, cheese, whole milk and butter): Dairy products too are known to have high fat contents. This said, low fat dairy products are not considered inflammatory.

Refined Carbohydrates (white bread, packaged cakes, and other pastries)

Margarine and coffee creamers: These items contain trans fats and there is no advisable or safe amount of this category to eat. The best thing is to avoid them.Pay close attention to whether they are list hydrogenated oils on their labels.

Deli meat: Processed meats such as deli meat have been noted to contain more glycation and products compared to other forms of meat. These are inflammatory compounds that form when meats are processed and cooked at high temperatures.

Canned soup: Perhaps make a homemade soup rather than relying on unhealthier, store-bought varieties. Most of the store bought soups on the market are associated with chronic inflammation. They are associated with diabetes and obesity.

Bacon: While bacon may taste great, it causes inflammation. The reasoning behind this is that bacon is highly saturated with fat, which results in increased inflammation in the body.

Vegetable and seed oils (sunflower, cottonseed, corn and soybean oil): It is true that some dietary omega-6 fats are necessary, however people tend to consume more omega-6 fats than needed. It is recommended that one create a balanced diet of omega-6 to omega-3 rations. Foods such as fish can provide this dietary need.

Sugar: The issue with sugar is that it causes inflammation throughout the body. Sugar, whether in the form of preservatives or dyes, causes inflammation.

White bread: Products like pastas and breads can quickly cause inflammation in the body. These are quickly digested by the body which leads to a rise of blood sugar levels. The result of this is that there is a spike in insulin which in turn leads to inflammation.

Drinks to Avoid

Excessive alcohol: An occasional glass of red wine is believed to be helpful in managing one's inflammation. Excessive alcohol though, is noted to be a trigger for inflammation. This is especially so for women, for whom drinking a glass of wine on a daily basis could result in leaky gut syndrome, which leads to total body inflammation.

Sweetened beverages such as soda: Soda is one of the most consumed drinks all over the world. It has been found that drinks with high sugar levels increase the occurrence of inflammation in a person's body.

Whole milk: A moderate intake of yogurt helps to reduce inflammation because it is capable of healing the gut. Dairy as a whole however is dense with saturated fats and act as a source of inflammation.

Inflammation FAQs

Q. Why does inflammation hurt?

The pain of inflammation is caused by tissue swelling and pressing on nerves.Also inflammation involves chemical substances changing molecular signals into an electric impulse that travels through the body, creating the sensation of pain.

Q. What is systemic inflammation?

It is an inflammation caused by the immune system to attack healthy tissues in the body. Systemic inflammation could become quite severe and if not checked and treated, result in organ failure or death.

Q. What is the relation between the immune system and inflammation?

The immune system could be sufficiently described as the protector of the body from harm by invaders. Whenever it senses danger, be it in the form of an injury or disease-causing bacteria, the immune system sends out its resources to attack the invader. When the immune system responds in this way, actually sending out white blood cells to fight the problem, soreness occurs. The variable in this relationship is that while sometimes these protective tools are needed by the body, in other instances they are not needed.

Q. Does inflammation synonymously identify with infection?

No, these two words do not mean the same thing. They may be confusing because they are closely related. However, whilst infection identifies as the body's occupation by foreign invaders, inflammation identifies as the process through which the body strives to fend off the invading foreigners.

Q. Is there medication to treat inflammation?

Yes, there are forms of inflammation that can be treated with various medications. Such substances as steroids and non-steroidal anti-inflammatory drugs (NSAIDs) are able to treat inflammatory.

Q. Does inflammation influence other diseases?

Yes. Inflammation is associated with a broad range of diseases such as asthma, heart disease and cancer, among others.

Q. What is "shock?"

Shock is defined as a "circulatory collapse", a condition where the body's blood pressure is low, hindering sufficient and free flow of blood throughout the body. The symptoms of this condition include dilated pupils, dry mouth, irregular breathing, quickened pulse and increased perspiration.

Q. Are organic meats or eggs less inflammatory?

Poultry and meat that have been raised on organic feed, free of antibiotics or hormones could be more nutritious. The challenge is a lack of nutritional data on these foods and the variety between the producers.

Q. Does a person who does not suffer from allergies or arthritis need to worry about inflammation?

Every person should worry about inflammation because it can happen to anyone, for a number of reasons. Inflammation can cause obvious symptoms such as asthma and joint pain.

Q. How does one know how to tell which foods are inflammatory?

It is complicated to distinguish foods that are inflammatory from foods that are anti-inflammatory. This is because some foods actually come with a combination of anti-inflammatory and inflammatory effects. The best motto is to research, practice and experiment!

As we already discussed, there are numerous benefits in following the Anti-inflammatory diet. Professionals and experts suggest following the Anti-inflammatory diet without giving it a second thought. However, before you start, there are a few rules that you must follow, which will be discussed below:

- Your primary focus should be on plant-based foods, including vegetables, fruits, whole grains, nuts, and legumes.
- You must replace butter with olive oil or other healthy oils.
- You must opt for spices and herbs instead of salt.
- You must add poultry and fish to your diet at least two times a week.
- You must limit red meat consumption, and eat only on special occasions or a few times a month.

- You must drink a lot of water and steer clear of unhealthy drinks. You can enjoy red wine in moderation.
- You must engage in exercise.
- Eat with your family and friends.

All these factors are essential because together, they will support your overall health. For example, eating with friends and family might not be outlined as a rule in any other diets, but in the Anti-inflammatory diet it is. Why do you think it is essential to dine with friends or family? Eating with family and friends will allow you to enjoy the food even more. You can test this out and see for yourself.

Traditionally, the Anti-inflammatory diet consists of pasta, rice, fruits, and vegetables. If you study the lifestyle of people in the Mediterranean region, you will understand their eating habits and why these foods are included in the diet. Even the grains in that region are whole grains and therefore have less trans fats. Bread is especially considered a vital part of this diet. When eating bread, it is essential not to apply margarine or butter to it because they contain trans fats, which is what we're trying to stay away from. Instead, you should coat the bread with olive oil. Nuts are an integral part of the diet too. You don't have to worry about the high calories in nuts because they are not saturated fats. When eating nuts, you shouldn't exceed the limit; simply try to limit your intake to a specified amount (maybe a handful of nuts) per day. You cannot substitute regular nuts for other nuts such as honey-roasted, salted, and candied. If you do, they will no longer fall under the allowed list of foods in the Anti-inflammatory diet.

As you already know, the Anti-inflammatory diet isn't entirely focused on fat consumption. Both hydrogenated oils and saturated fats are not encouraged in the Anti-inflammatory diet because they can lead to the development of heart disease.

Olive oil is considered the best type of oil that can be consumed in the Anti-inflammatory diet, as it has monounsaturated fats; therefore, it reduces the levels of LDL cholesterol. Both virgin and extra-virgin olive oils are processed in the lowest form. They contain antioxidants which are needed for the body. Linolenic acid is found in polyunsaturated fats and monounsaturated fats. Omega-3 fatty acids help to reduce triglycerides and blood clotting. They will enhance the health of the blood vessels as well. You can eat fish regularly, as well as fatty fish including lake trout, sardines, mackerel, salmon, and tuna, as they are enriched with omega-3 fatty acids.

Alcohol is not recommended by the Anti-inflammatory diet. There has been an ongoing debate about whether or not alcohol consumption should be permitted in this diet. Some professionals don't allow the consumption of alcohol, however, wine consumption is allowed if the dieter only moderately consumes it. Women are allowed to consume around 148 milliliters of wine, which is five ounces per day. Men (under the age of 65) are allowed to consume around 296 milliliters, which adds up to ten ounces per day. If you are someone who has little control over consumption of wine or alcohol, it's best to stay away from it altogether. This way, you will be able to control your cravings, and opt for something else instead.

It can be tough to get started on this type of diet, even if you know what to eat and what to avoid. But if you can find a way to create a specialized meal plan, you will be able to move forward with ease. Below I've outlined a few steps that you should follow if you want to get started with this type of diet.

Find solutions for snacks: At some point, you will want to grab a quick snack, so what kind of snacks are you allowed to have? Some snacks you're allowed to eat are cashews, almonds, walnuts, pistachios, and even non hydrogenated peanut butter. You can easily prepare these snacks in an instant. Just remember to keep your snacking habits at a healthy level.

Have more fruits and veggies: In the past, vegetables may not have been your favorite, but if they can improve your overall health, you should add them to your diet plan. Try to include whole grains, fruits, and veggies as much as possible. Your meals should have a high percentage of plant-based foods. It's best to have around

7-10 servings of fruits or vegetables per day. You should also consider whole-grain products such as pasta and rice.

Ditch the butter: Butter is not necessary if you have canola or olive oil because they will serve the same purpose as butter would.

Add fish: Add tuna, mackerel, trout, and other healthy choices of fish to your diet. If you are interested in fried fish, you should first make sure you use the right type of oil, such as olive oil or canola oil.

Opt for spices and herbs: If you have been using salt, it is time to switch to spices and herbs because they promote health and are delicious.

Consider low-fat diary: Opt for products that are low in fat like fat-free cheese, yogurt, and skim milk. Stay away from dairy products that have a high fat percentage.

The above list is important, and you should familiarize yourself with it before starting your journey on the Anti-inflammatory diet. Below, I've gone into more detail about the foods you can and cannot have with this diet.

Foods to Eat When on the Anti-Inflammatory Diet

Vegetables: kale, broccoli, tomatoes, onions, cauliflower, spinach, carrots, cucumbers, Brussels sprouts, etc.

Fruits: grapes, bananas, apples, pears, oranges, dates, melons, figs, peaches, strawberries, etc.

Legumes: chickpeas, peanuts, lentils, peas, beans, pulses, etc.

Nuts: walnuts, almonds, hazelnuts, macadamia nuts, cashews, pumpkin seeds, sunflower seeds, etc.

Whole grains: brown rice, whole oats, barley, rye, corn, whole wheat, buckwheat, pasta, and whole-grain bread.

Tubers: turnip, yams, potatoes, and sweet potatoes.

Seafood and fish: oysters, shrimp, mackerel, sardines, crabs, clams, mussels, salmon, etc.

Eggs: duck, chicken, and quail eggs.

Low-fat dairy: low-fat cheese, Greek yogurt, etc.

Poultry: duck, chicken, turkey, etc.

Spices and herbs: basil, garlic, mint, sage, rosemary, cinnamon, nutmeg, pepper, etc.

Healthy fats: avocado oil, Extra-virgin olive oil, etc.

Foods to Avoid When on the Anti-Inflammatory Diet

Added sugar: ice cream, candies, table sugar, and soda.

Trans fat: fats that are in processed foods and margarine.

Refined grains: refined wheat products, white bread, etc.

Refined oils: canola oil, soybean oil, cottonseed oil, etc.

Processed meat: hot dogs, sausages, etc.

Highly processed foods: Make sure to check the packaging to ensure whether or not the food is highly processed. It is essential to read labels so that you can find out whether the ingredients are healthy or not.

Even if this takes time, don't rush. Your health is important.

What to Drink When on the Anti-inflammatory Diet

As you already know, water should become your favorite beverage when you are on the Anti-inflammatory diet. As mentioned earlier, you can drink red wine too, but you should set yourself a limit to how much you can drink. If you are struggling with alcoholism, you should avoid wine completely. You can drink tea and coffee instead, but without added sugar. You should also avoid fruit juice beverages as well.

It is not easy to adopt a new diet in just a day or two. However, give it a try anyway. You won't know what it's like unless you try.

Chapter 7: 2-Week Diet Plan

Now, we've reached the vital part of the book, which is the 14-Days Meal Plan. In this section of the book, I've included a number of delicious recipes that you can make in less than 20 minutes.

Mediterranean Breakfast Recipes
Scrambled Eggs with Spinach and Raspberries

Time needed: 10 minutes

Servings: 1

This is a quick recipe that you can prepare in a short amount of time, that will turn out delicious. This dish combines filling and weight-loss based ingredients. You'll be energized the rest of your day if you have this breakfast.

Ingredients:

1 teaspoon olive oil

1 ½ cups baby spinach

2 large eggs (slightly beaten)

1 slice whole-grain bread

½ cup toasted raspberries

Pinch of black pepper and kosher salt

How to Prepare:

- Take a small skillet (non-stick).
- Set it over medium-high heat and add oil.
- Stir in spinach and let it cook for 1-2 minutes.
- Transfer the cooked spinach to a container.
- In the same pan, add eggs while setting the medium heat.
- Stir, and check whether it's cooked, and let it remain for 2 minutes.
- Add the cooked spinach, black pepper, and kosher salt.
- Finally, enjoy scrambled eggs with toast and raspberries.

Macros:

296 calories

18 grams protein

16 grams fat

21 grams carbohydrates

Tomato, Cucumber, and Feta Salad

Time needed: 10 minutes

Servings: 4

This is an ideal Mediterranean salad that is enriched with a lot of flavor. This delicious dish can be prepared in as short as 10 minutes. You can also serve this dish with some grilled fish.

Ingredients:

1 ½ tablespoon red-wine vinegar

1 teaspoon fresh oregano (chopped)

Oregano leaves (for garnish)

½ teaspoon Dijon mustard

¼ teaspoon Kosher salt

3 tablespoons Extra-virgin olive oil

4 sliced crosswise Persian cucumber

2 cups (8 ounces) Campari tomatoes (wedges)

1 ½ ounce Feta cheese (crumbled)

How to prepare:

Take a medium-size bowl.

Whisk oregano, vinegar, salt, and mustard together.

Drizzle olive oil and whisk steadily.

Then, add cucumbers, feta cheese, tomatoes, and mix.

If preferred, garnish using the small oregano leaves.

For better taste, serve right away.

Recipe notes:

1. If you can't find Persian cucumber and Campari tomatoes, you can opt for any other cucumbers or tomatoes, but note that there will be changes in the macros.
2. If you are meal prepping, prepare the dressing ahead, transfer it to an airtight container, and refrigerate it so that you can use it when you are prepared to eat.

3. You can refrigerate this dish for up to three days.

Macros:

153 calories

3 grams protein

13 grams fat

6 grams carbohydrates

Avocado and Apple Smoothie

Time needed: 15 minutes

Servings: 2

Smoothies are a great go-to breakfast option for busy individuals. Green smoothies are not only delicious, but also healthy! This breakfast will detoxify your body, and will make you feel great.

Ingredients:

1 cup unsweetened almond milk

4 cups spinach

1 medium apple (peeled and quartered)

1 avocado (peeled and pitted)

1 banana (cut into chunks and frozen)

2 teaspoons honey

½ teaspoon ground ginger

Ice cubes

Almond butter, flaxseed, or chia seeds (optional)

How to prepare:

1. Take a high-powered blender.
2. Add almond milk, avocado, spinach, apples, honey, banana, ginger, ice cubes, and honey.
3. Blend the ingredients until smooth.
4. Taste and add spices and sweetness if needed.
5. Enjoy right away.

Recipe notes:

1. You can store the leftovers in an airtight container and refrigerate them for a day. Or you can halve the ingredients if the smoothie is for one person.
2. If you don't own a high-powered blender, you should blend the spinach, avocado, and almond

milk separately first. Then, add banana, apple, ginger, and honey.

3. Once you get a smooth texture, add ice cubes.

Macros:

306 calories

4 grams protein

13 grams fat

15 grams carbohydrates

Cucumber and Heirloom Tomato Toast

Time needed: 5 minutes

Servings: 1

Find the freshest and ripest ingredients to prepare this toast, and make it a delicious meal. You can make this dish in just five minutes, and it can be considered a great breakfast, dinner, or lunch meal; the choice is yours!

Ingredients:

1 small heirloom tomato (diced)

1 Persian cucumber (diced)

Pinch of oregano (dried)

1 teaspoon Extra-virgin oil

2 teaspoons whipped cream cheese (low-fat)

2 pieces whole grain bread

1 teaspoon balsamic glaze

Black pepper and kosher salt

How to prepare:

- Take a medium bowl.
- Add in cucumber, tomato, oregano, olive oil and toss.
- Then, season with black pepper and kosher salt.
- Apply the cream cheese on the whole grain bread and add the salad on top with some balsamic glaze.

Macros:

177 calories

3 grams protein

8 grams fat

24 grams carbohydrates

Time needed: 10 minutes

Servings: 4

Normally this salad is made with grilled steak, but with this recipe try it out with some grilled halloumi instead. This delicious and easy to make meal can be made in just 10 minutes.

Ingredients:

1 pound tomatoes (sliced in circular shapes)

½ pound Halloumi cheese (four slabs)

½ lemon

Extra-virgin olive oil (as needed)

5 basil leaves (torn)

2 tablespoons parsley leaves (finely chopped)

Ground pepper and kosher salt

How to prepare:

1. Begin by preheating the grill and setting it to medium-high.
2. Next, place the tomatoes on four plates and squeeze the lemon over them. Also, season with ground pepper and kosher salt.
3. Once the grill is oiled, place the halloumi and let it cook. Make sure to flip sides and ensure it's cooked properly.
4. Spend around 1 minute on each side of the halloumi, or until you notice grill marks.
5. Place the finished halloumi on top of the neatly arranged tomatoes, drizzle olive oil and add parsley and basil.
6. Enjoy!

Macros:

196 calories

9 grams protein

15 grams fat

8 grams carbohydrates

Pasta with Lemon Basil Shrimp

Time needed: 20 minutes

Servings: 4

This recipe is one of the most straightforward recipes that you can prepare in just twenty minutes. Shrimp can make any dish mouth-watering; especially if you love seafood. Lemon and basil will give the final touch to this meal! This high protein meal will also keep you energized throughout the day.

Ingredients:

3 quarts water

8 ounces uncooked spaghetti

1 pound large shrimp (peeled and deveined)

¼ cup fresh basil (chopped)

3 tablespoons drained capers

2 cups baby spinach

2 tablespoons Extra-virgin olive oil

2 tablespoons lemon juice

½ teaspoon Kosher salt

How to prepare:

- Begin by bringing the water to a boil in a Dutch oven.
- Next, stir in the pasta and cook for about 8 minutes.
- Then, take a pan and set it over medium heat.
- Add shrimp and let it cook for about 3 minutes.
- Meanwhile, check the pasta and if it's done, drain it.
- Shift the pasta to a large bowl.
- Add basil, lemon juice, drained capers, olive oil, and kosher salt to the bowl.
- Take four plates and serve spinach on each (½ cup per plate) and pasta mixture (1 ½ cups).
- Add the cooked shrimp on top and enjoy!

Macros:

397 calories

31 grams protein

9.6 grams fat

44.9 grams carbohydrates

Pepperoncini, Tuna with Couscous

Time needed: 15 minutes

Servings: 4

It's important to treat yourself to a fancy meal every now and then, right? Pepperoncini, tuna with couscous is a fancy meal that you can prepare in just 15 minutes. This meal is filled with flavorful ingredients that will ensure you have an enjoyable and delicious meal.

Ingredients for couscous:

1 ¼ cups couscous

1 cup water or chicken broth

¾ teaspoon Kosher salt

Ingredients for accompaniments:

2 cans (5 ounces) oil-packed tuna

1 pint cherry tomatoes (halved)

½ cup pepperoncini (sliced)

⅓ cup fresh parsley (chopped)

¼ cup capers

Extra-virgin olive oil (for serving)

1 Lemon (quartered)

Ground pepper and kosher salt

How to prepare:

1. Begin by preparing the couscous.
2. Take a small pot and set over medium heat.
3. Bring the water or chicken broth to a boil.
4. Switch off the heat and add couscous and cover with a lid. Let it remain covered for about 10 minutes.
5. Next, prepare the accompaniments.
6. Take a medium-size bowl and add the tomatoes, tuna, parsley, capers, and pepperoncini together.
7. Use a fork to fluff the prepared couscous and season it with pepper, salt, and olive oil.
8. Before serving, add tuna mixture on top along with lemon wedges.

Macros (couscous)

226 calories

8 grams protein

1 grams fat

44 grams carbohydrates

Macros (accompaniments)

193 calories

22 grams protein

9 grams fat

6 grams carbohydrates

Toasted Za'atar Pita Bread with Mezze Plate

Time needed: 15 minutes

Servings: 2

This recipe is as exciting as its name. There's no doubt that you'll keep wanting more of this dish. The delicious herbed pitas are what make this dish so wonderful. Moreover, no cooking is required to prepare this recipe.

Ingredients:

4 rounds whole-wheat pita

4 teaspoons za'atar

4 tablespoons extra-virgin olive oil

1 cup Greek yogurt

1 cup hummus

1 cup marinated artichoke hearts

1 cup red peppers (sliced and roasted)

2 cups cherry tomatoes

2 cups assorted olives

4 ounces salami

Kosher salt and black pepper

How to prepare:

1. Take a large skillet and place it on medium-high heat.
2. Add olive oil to either side of the pitas and drizzle with za'atar.
3. Cook in batches.

4. Place pitas on the heated skillet and let it toast for about 2 minutes on each side.
5. Then, quarter each pita.
6. Next, sprinkle some pepper and salt on the Greek yogurt.
7. Finally, assemble your dish by dividing the pitas, hummus, artichoke hearts, Greek yogurt, olives, red peppers, salami, and tomatoes onto four plates.

Macros:

731 calories

26 grams protein

48 grams fat

62 grams carbohydrates

The Cold Lemon Zucchini

Time needed: 20 minutes

Servings: 4

This dish is an enjoyable cold meal. This dish gives you the option to have something cold on days where the heat is too much to handle. This recipe is simple to prepare.

Ingredients:

1 lemon (zested and juiced)

½ teaspoon Dijon mustard

½ teaspoon garlic powder

⅓ cup Olive oil

1 bunch radishes (thinly sliced)

1 tablespoon fresh thyme (chopped)

3 medium zucchinis (cut into noodles)

Kosher salt and black pepper

How to prepare:

1. Take a bowl and whisk the lemon juice and zest, garlic powder, and mustard together.
2. Slowly, add olive oil and mix. Season with pepper and salt.

3. Meanwhile, take a large bowl and add the radishes and zucchini noodles. Then, add the prepared dressing. Make sure to toss until well coated.
4. Enjoy immediately by garnishing with thyme.

Macros:

198 calories

2 grams protein

19 grams fat

8 grams net carbohydrates

Roasted Red Pepper Pauce and Mediterranean Quinoa Dish

Time needed: 20 minutes

Servings: 8

It's time to wave goodbye to time-consuming meal preparations. This lunch recipe is a special one. It's also a great recipe for holiday parties. You'll be saving a lot of time and energy preparing this dish. It only takes 20 minutes to prepare it.

Ingredients for the Mediterranean bowls:

Quinoa (cooked)

Feta cheese

Cucumber, spinach, or kale

Kalamata olives

Red onion (thinly sliced)

Pepperoncini

Hummus

Parsley or fresh basil

Salt, pepper, lemon juice, and olive oil

Ingredients roasted red pepper sauce:

½ cup Olive oil

1 garlic clove

½ cup almonds

1 16 ounce jar roasted red peppers (drained)

½ teaspoon salt

1 lemon (juiced)

How to prepare:

1. With a blender of food processor, add all the ingredients needed to prepare the sauce. Pulse it until you get a thick texture.
2. To prepare the quinoa, read the instructions on the package. Once done, arrange the Mediterranean quinoa bowl to your preference.
3. Enjoy with the prepared sauce.

Recipe notes:

1. To cook the quinoa, you can use a rice cooker while you prepare everything else.
2. If you are a vegetarian, you can exchange the feta cheese for white beans.
3. Use plastic containers to store away any leftovers.

Macros:

381 calories

10.9 grams protein

25.6 grams fat

30.9 grams net carbohydrates

Avocado Dressing-Added Chickpea and Kale Grain Bowl

Time needed: 20 minutes

Servings: 4

This particular salad bowl is filled with a number of colorful and flavorful ingredients. All the ingredients together will make it a great bowl, however, it's the avocado dressing which will add the final touch to it. It will not only add color to your salad but also a number of health benefits. This veggie bowl will help with digestion, and provide you with energy throughout the day. This is one of the best Mediterranean salads that you can prepare in a short time.

Ingredients:

1 cup boiling water

½ cup uncooked bulgur

1 ½ tablespoons olive oil

2 cans (15 ounces) chickpeas (unsalted, rinsed, and drained)

2 cups carrots (finely chopped)

½ cup shallots (vertically sliced)

4 cups lacinato kale (chopped)

½ cup parsley leaves (flat-leaf)

½ avocado (peeled and pitted)

1 garlic clove

1 tablespoon tahini (sesame seed paste)

½ teaspoon black pepper

¾ teaspoon Kosher salt

2 tablespoons extra-virgin olive oil

1 tablespoon lemon juice

1 tablespoon water

¼ teaspoon ground turmeric

How to prepare:

1. Take a medium-sized bowl and add in the bulgur and boiling water.Mix together for 10 minutes and drain.
2. Using paper towels, dry the chickpeas.
3. Meanwhile, place a skillet over high heat and add the olive oil.
4. Then, add carrots and chickpeas to the skillet and cook. Make sure to stir often. Let it cook for 6 minutes.
5. Add kale and cover the skillet. Wait around 2 minutes, or until wilted.
6. Stir chickpea mixture, parsley, shallots, pepper, and salt to the prepared bulgur and mix.
7. To make the avocado dressing, in a food processor, add olive oil, water, lemon juice, garlic, tahini, turmeric, and remaining salt.
8. Process until you get the smooth texture.
9. Divide bulgur equally among four bowls and drizzle the avocado mixture over top.

Macros:

520 calories

18 grams protein

20 grams fat

68 grams carbohydrates

Pasta Salad with Eggplant and Tomatoes

Time needed: 20 minutes

Servings: 4

This is a filling salad that will leave you feeling satiated. It's normally not easy to feel satiated with just a bowl of salad, but this one is an exception because of its filling and delicious ingredients.

Ingredients:

8 ounces uncooked casarecce

1 tablespoon olive oil

2 cups eggplant (chopped)

¼ cup dry white wine

1 tablespoon garlic (minced)

2 pints cherry tomatoes (halved)

2 teaspoons white wine vinegar

2 teaspoons fresh thyme (chopped)

½ teaspoon Kosher salt

6 ounces burrata

½ teaspoon black pepper

How to prepare:

1. Read the directions on the package and cook the pasta accordingly.
2. In the last 3 minutes, add beans to the pasta. Drain the pasta and set aside a cup of cooking liquid from the pasta.
3. Meanwhile, take a large skillet and place it over medium-high heat.
4. Stir in eggplant and cook while stirring occasionally. Stir for around 4-5 minutes, until tender.
5. Stir in garlic and cook for 1 minute, then, stir in half of the cherry tomatoes. Cook for about 2-3 minutes.
6. Next, add the wine and stir.

7. Stir in beans and pasta. Mix well. Now, add in a tablespoon of the cooking liquid you set aside.
8. Add the remaining tomatoes, salt, and vinegar.
9. Take four bowls and serve the pasta into the bowls.
10. Top with thyme, pepper, and burrata.

Recipe notes:

If you don't have burrata, you can add 6 ounces of mozzarella and chop it into bite size pieces.

Macros:

428 calories

17 grams protein

14 grams fat

56 grams carbohydrates

Cucumber and Chicken Salad Along with Parsley Pesto

Time needed: 15 minutes

Servings: 6

This hearty salad is filled with lean-protein, thanks to chickpeas, chicken, and edamame. If you don't have a lot of time and wish to prepare to salad even faster, you could use frozen edamame.

Ingredients:

1 cup baby spinach

2 cups flat-leaf parsley leaves

1 tablespoon pine nuts (toasted)

2 tablespoons fresh lemon juice

1 tablespoon Parmesan cheese (grated)

1 garlic clove (medium and smashed)

½ cup Extra-virgin olive oil

4 cups rotisserie chicken (shredded)

2 cups shelled edamame (cooked)

1 can (15 ounces) chickpeas (unsalted, drained and rinsed)

1 cup English cucumber (chopped)

4 cups loosely packed arugula

1 teaspoon Kosher salt

¼ teaspoon black pepper

How to prepare:

1. Grab a food processor and add in spinach, parsley, lemon juice, cheese, pine nuts, salt, garlic, and pepper.
2. Process for about 1 minute and check whether it is a smooth texture.
3. While the processor runs, add in the oil and stir for one minute.
4. Take a large bowl and add the edamame, chicken, cucumber, and chickpeas.
5. Divide arugula into six bowls (⅔ cup per bowl).
6. Then, add a cup of chicken salad mixture to all six bowls on top of the arugula.
7. Enjoy!

Macros:

482 calories

40 grams protein

26 grams fat

22 grams carbohydrates

Mediterranean Snack Recipes
Carrot Cake Bites

Time *needed*: 15 minutes

Servings: 30-40 (varies as per the size you make)

Carrot cake bites are the best when you want something to snack on. These little snacks are so delicious that you might never stop snacking on them.

Ingredients:

1 medium carrot (peeled and chopped)

½ cup almond butter

½ cup pure maple syrup

2 cups unsweetened flaked coconut

2 cups old fashioned oats

½ teaspoon vanilla

½ teaspoon Kosher salt

1 teaspoon cinnamon

Chocolate chips (optional)

How to prepare:

- Begin by cutting the carrot into chunks and then, add the chunks to a food processor. Pulse until chopped.
- Keep aside chopped carrots, and add the coconut and oats. Pulse until chopped.
- Then, add all the ingredients together and pulse until smooth. Use a spatula to combine all the ingredients if they stick to the processor bowl.
- Add in chocolate chips; pulse once again.
- Now, you can prepare the balls and freeze.

Macros:

87 calories

1.8 grams protein

5 grams fat

9.2 grams carbohydrates

Quick Vegan Yogurt

Time needed: 5 minutes

Servings: 4

Homemade anything is always fun, and so is this homemade yogurt! Prepare this vegan yogurt with just three ingredients while sweetening it naturally.

Ingredients:

½ cup cashews

2 cups frozen peaches

12 ounces tofu

1 tablespoon lemon juice

¼ cup liquid sweetener (agave, maple syrup, honey)

1 probiotic capsule (optional)

How to prepare:

- Add all the ingredients together and blend on high speed. Blend until smooth.

- Enjoy!

Recipe notes:

You can store this yogurt in the fridge for up to 5 days.

If you find it hard to blend the ingredients together, you can add ¼-½ cup of non-dairy milk. To blend easily, thaw frozen peaches first.

If you want the probiotic boost, you can add a probiotic capsule to the mixture. Remove the cover and add the powder to the mixture. Adding the probiotic capsule is always optional.

Macros:

262 calories

18 grams protein

12.4 grams fat

32.2 grams carbohydrates

Two-Minute Avocado Dip

Time needed: 2 minutes

Servings: 2

Avocado dip goes well with almost any variety of chips. Plus, it's also healthy. You can prepare avocado dip in as little as two minutes!

Ingredients:

1 avocado

¼ cup plain Greek yogurt

Lime juice to taste

¼ teaspoon salt

Pinch of garlic powder

How to prepare:

1. Begin by mashing the avocado.
2. Add in the lime juice, yogurt, salt, and garlic powder.
3. Taste and adjust accordingly! Yes, simple as that.

Recipe notes:

Add chopped cilantro if you wish, or add cayenne or jalapeno to spice it up.

Macros:

155 calories

4.7 grams protein

12.3 grams fat

9.4 grams carbohydrates

Mediterranean Dinner Recipes
Sweet Potato Noodles and Almond Sauce

Time needed: 20 minutes

Servings: 4

If you have been looking for delicious vegan dinner recipes for a while now, this is one of them. This recipe is filling and full of texture. It's also packed with a number of vitamins and proteins, making it a healthy meal.

Ingredients for Almond sauce:

2 tablespoons extra-virgin olive oil

3 shallots (minced)

2 garlic cloves (minced)

2 cups unsweetened almond milk

3 tablespoons all-purpose flour

2 tablespoons Dijon mustard

Salt and black pepper

Ingredients for Sweet potato noodles:

2 tablespoons extra-virgin olive oil

3 sweet potatoes (cut into noodles)

4 cups torn kale

½ cup almonds (toasted and chopped)

Salt and black pepper

How to prepare:

1. Begin by making the almond sauce. Take a medium-sized pot, add olive oil and place over medium heat.
2. Stir in garlic and shallots; sauté for one minute.
3. Add flour and cook for one minute.
4. Next, pour almond milk and mix to avoid lumps. Let it simmer for 4-5 minutes.

5. Add Dijon mustard and flavor the almond sauce with pepper and salt. Cover and reduce the heat.
6. Use a spiralizer to make noodles out of the sweet potatoes.
7. Take a large pan, add olive oil, and place it over medium heat.
8. Then, add in the noodles and stir occasionally. Wait 4-5 minutes or until tender.
9. Toss in the kale and sauce. Make sure the noodles are well coated.
10. Season the mixture with pepper and salt.
11. Add the almonds and serve.

Macros Almond Sauce:

139 calories

3 grams protein

8 grams fat

14 grams carbohydrates

Macros Sweet Potato Noodles:

256 calories

6 grams protein

16 grams fat

25 grams carbohydrates

Courgette, Shaved Fennel, and Orange Salad

Time needed: 15 minutes

Servings: 4

It's always enjoyable to eat a fresh salad. This recipe might be one of the most straightforward recipes for a salad you will ever make.

Ingredients:

1 orange

2 small fennel bulbs

1 baby gem lettuce (washed and leaves separated)

2 small courgettes (green or yellow)

2 teaspoons sherry vinegar

4 tablespoons olive oil

½ cup lemon juice

How to prepare:

1. Peel the orange.
2. Cut the slices of the orange into halves. You can keep the juice collected from the orange as dressing.
3. Take a bowl and stir all the ingredients together.
4. Clean the fennel thoroughly, halve it, and cut the cores out. Then, slice the fennel into thin pieces.
5. Cut the ends of the courgettes with the help of a peeler.
6. Add in the orange juice that you kept aside, olive oil, and sherry vinegar to the same bowl.
7. Toss the mixture together so that everything combines well.
8. Before serving, add the mixed courgette, lettuce leaves, fennel, and orange slices together.

Macros:

170 calories

3 grams protein

12 grams fat

25 grams carbohydrates

Easy Mediterranean Fish Meal

Time needed: 20 minutes

Servings: 4

If you are looking for an easy-to-make meal with fish, this recipe is the one for you. You can make this meal with the available ingredients in your kitchen, so you don't have to go out and buy any special ingredients.

Ingredients:

1 tablespoon almond butter

1 pound white fish

12 ounce jar artichoke salad

1 cup fresh baby spinach (chopped)

⅓ cup sundried tomatoes (chopped)

1 teaspoon garlic (crushed)

2 tablespoons capers

How to prepare:

1. Begin by thawing the fish if frozen.
2. Take the sauté pan and melt almond butter by setting it to medium-high heat.
3. Add fish and cook for about 2 minutes on each side.
4. Then, stir in all the ingredients and cook for 10 minutes at medium heat.
5. You can enjoy it as it is or with some cauliflower rice!

Macros:

325 calories

34.2 grams protein

16.6 grams fat

12.3 grams carbohydrates

Mango Pineapple Salsa with Cajun Mahi Mahi

Time needed: 15 minutes

Servings: 4

This recipe is different from the rest. It is also probably a recipe you wouldn't normally make. I can assure you though that you will love its taste. The pineapple salsa makes this recipe that much better.

Ingredients for Cajun Mahi Mahi:

1.5 pound of fresh Mahi Mahi fillets

1 tablespoon Cajun spice seasoning

½ tablespoon garlic powder

2 tablespoons grapeseed oil

Ingredients Mango Pineapple Salsa:

1 mango (finely diced)

1 cup pineapple (fresh diced)

¼ cup red onion (finely diced)

¼ cup fresh cilantro (chopped)

1-2 tablespoons lime juice

Kosher salt

How to prepare:

1. Take a small bowl and add the mango, fresh cilantro, pineapple, salt, and lime juice. Mix everything and keep it aside.
2. In another bowl, add in cajun spice and garlic powder and mix.
3. Dry the Mahi Mahi fillets.
4. Season the Mahi Mahi fillets using cajun seasoning mixture.
5. Heat a skillet to medium-high heat. Then, heat the grapeseed oil.
6. Sear the Mahi Mahi fillets for 2-3 minutes on each side.
7. Remove from the stove and let it sit for a minute.
8. Enjoy!

Macros:

175 calories

22 grams protein

6 grams fat

11 grams carbohydrates

Cauliflower Rice

Time needed: 20 minutes

Servings: 4

This recipe is similar to fried rice, only it is a much healthier alternative.

Ingredients:

5 cups (24 ounces) cauliflower florets

2 tablespoons of reduced sodium soy sauce

1 tablespoon sesame oil

1 tablespoon ginger (grated)

2 tablespoons vegetable oil

2 green onions (thinly sliced)

2 large eggs

¼ teaspoon white pepper

6 ounces broccoli florets (chopped)

2 garlic cloves (minced)

1 onion (diced)

2 carrots (peeled and grated)

½ cup frozen peas

½ cup frozen corn

½ teaspoon sesame seeds

How to prepare:

1. Before making the cauliflower rice, you must use a food processor to pulse the cauliflower so that it turns into rice. Pulse it for around 3 minutes and set aside.
2. Take a bowl and whisk the sesame oil, soy sauce, white pepper, ginger, and place it aside.
3. Then, take a medium-sized skillet and heat a tablespoon of oil and set it to low heat. Add in the eggs and cook for about 3 minutes on each side.
4. Next, add the remaining oil to the skillet and place over medium-high heat. Add onion and garlic to it and occasionally stir. Cook for 3-4 minutes. Add corn, carrots, broccoli, and peas and stir occasionally. Wait 3-4 minutes, or until vegetables are tender.

5. Add eggs, cauliflower, soy sauce, and green onions. Cook for 4 minutes while stirring occasionally, until cauliflower is tender.
6. Garnish the finished product with sesame seeds and serve.

Macros:

252.9 calories

10.6 grams protein

13.8 grams fat

26.8 grams carbohydrates

Spicy Shrimp, Garlic Kale with Cauliflower Mash

Time needed: 20 minutes

Servings: 4

This recipe is quick and easy to make. It could even become your favorite weeknight dinner recipe. It also only takes up 20 minutes of your time.

Ingredients for the cauliflower mash:

1 tablespoon olive oil

1 head cauliflower (chopped)

3 garlic cloves (minced)

1 cup milk

3 cups chicken or vegetable broth

1 14-ounce can white beans (rinsed and drained)

½ cup cornmeal

½ cup shredded cheese

1 teaspoon salt

Ingredients for the kale:

1 tablespoon bacon fat

3 cups of chopped kale

3 garlic cloves (minced)

Ingredient for the shrimp:

1 tablespoon olive oil

1 pound shrimp

Chile powder

Garlic salt

Black pepper

Cayenne

How to prepare:

1. Prepare the cauliflower. Take a large pot and heat the oil. Add the garlic and the cauliflower.
2. Saute for 1-2 minutes. Then, add broth and milk and let simmer for 10 minutes. Next, add the beans. Use a wooden spoon to mash the mixture until chunky.
3. Add cornmeal to make the mixture thick. You can balance the consistency with the available cup of broth. But do it only if needed. Add cheese and salt to taste.
4. Next, prepare the kale. Take a nonstick skillet and place over medium-low heat. Add the bacon fat, let it heat. Next, saute the garlic and greens. Add a little bit of water for the kale to steam. Once done, remove the kale and clean the pan.
5. Finally, prepare the shrimp. You can use the same skillet as before. Heat the pan and add oil to it.

After drying the shrimp, you can add them to the skillet. Drizzle the seasoning accordingly. Then, cook for a few minutes and add broth or water to the skillet (approximately 2 tablespoons).

6. That's it! Enjoy your shrimp and kale with cauliflower mash.

Macros:

409 calories

34.7 grams protein

16.5 grams fat

32.3 grams carbohydrates

Day 1

Breakfast: Scrambled eggs with spinach and raspberries

Macro nutrition information

Carbohydrates— 21 grams

Fat— 16 grams

Protein— 18 grams

Kcal— 296

Lunch: Grilled halloumi, herbs, and tomato salad

Macro nutrition information

Carbohydrates— 8 grams

Fat— 15 grams

Protein— 9 grams

Kcal— 196

Dinner: Sweet Potato Noodles and Almond Sauce

Macro nutrition information

Carbohydrates— 39 grams

Fat— 24 grams

Protein— 9 grams

Kcal— 395

Total kcal for the day— 887

Day 2
Breakfast: Tomato, Cucumber and Feta Salad

Macro nutrition information

Carbohydrates— 6 grams

Fat— 13 grams

Protein— 3 grams

Kcal— 153

Lunch: Pasta with lemon basil shrimp

Macro nutrition information

Carbohydrates— 44.9 grams

Fat— 13 grams

Protein— 3 grams

Kcal— 153

Dinner: Basil Garlic Shrimp Farrotto

Macro nutrition information

Carbohydrates— 46.2 grams

Fat— 13.7 grams

Protein— 27.2 grams

Kcal— 415

Total kcal for the day— 721

Breakfast: Avocado and Apple Smoothie

Macro nutrition information

Carbohydrates— 15 grams

Fat— 13 grams

Protein— 4 grams

Kcal— 306

Lunch: Pepperoncini, tuna with couscous

Macro nutrition information

Carbohydrates— 50 grams

Fat— 10 grams

Protein— 30 grams

Kcal— 419

Dinner: Easy Mediterranean Fish meal

Macro nutrition information

Carbohydrates— 12.3 grams

Fat— 16.6 grams

Protein— 34.2 grams

Kcal— 325

Total kcal for the day— 1, 050

Day 4
Breakfast: Cucumber and Heirloom Tomato Toast

Macro nutrition information

Carbohydrates— 24 grams

Fat— 8 grams

Protein— 3 grams

Kcal— 177

Lunch: Toasted Za'atar Pita Bread with Mezze Plate

Macro nutrition information

Carbohydrates— 62 grams

Fat— 48 grams

Protein— 26 grams

Kcal— 731

Dinner: Mango Pineapple Salsa with Cajun Mahi Mahi

Macro nutrition information

Carbohydrates— 11 grams

Fat— 6 grams

Protein— 22 grams

Kcal— 175

Total kcal for the day— 1, 083

Day 5
Breakfast: Mediterranean Breakfast Couscous

Macro nutrition information

Carbohydrates— 55 grams

Fat— 6 grams

Protein— 11 grams

Kcal— 306

Lunch: Cold Lemon Zucchini

Macro nutrition information

Carbohydrates— 8 grams

Fat— 19 grams

Protein— 2 grams

Kcal— 198

Dinner: Cauliflower rice

Macro nutrition information

Carbohydrates— 26.8 grams

Fat— 13.8 grams

Protein— 10.6 grams

Kcal— 252.9

Total kcal for the day— 756.9

Day 6
Breakfast: Potato hash and chickpea recipe

Macro nutrition information

Carbohydrates— 37 grams

Fat— 20 grams

Protein— 14 grams

Kcal— 382

Lunch: Roasted red pepper sauce and Mediterranean quinoa dish

Macro nutrition information

Carbohydrates— 30.9 grams

Fat— 25.6 grams

Protein— 10.9 grams

Kcal— 381

Dinner: Spicy shrimp, Garlic Kale with cauliflower mash

Macro nutrition information

Carbohydrates— 32.3 grams

Fat— 16.5 grams

Protein— 34.7 grams

Kcal— 409

Total kcal for the day— 1,172

Day 7

Breakfast: Peanut Butter Protein Shake

Macro nutrition information

Carbohydrates— 41 grams

Fat— 16 grams

Protein— 26 grams

Kcal— 402

Lunch: Repeat meal from day 2

Macro nutrition information

Carbohydrates— 44.9 grams

Fat— 13 grams

Protein— 3 grams

Kcal— 153

Dinner: Repeat meal from day 3

Macro nutrition information

Carbohydrates— 12.3 grams

Fat— 16.6 grams

Protein— 34.2 grams

Kcal— 325

Total kcal for the day— 880

Day 8
Breakfast: Repeat meal from day 1

Macro nutrition information

Carbohydrates— 21 grams

Fat— 16 grams

Protein— 18 grams

Kcal— 296

Lunch: Mediterranean Lettuce Wraps

Macro nutrition information

Carbohydrates— 44 grams

Fat— 28 grams

Protein— 16 grams

Kcal— 498

Dinner: Repeat meal from day 1

Macro nutrition information

Carbohydrates— 39 grams

Fat— 24 grams

Protein— 9 grams

Kcal— 395

Total kcal for the day— 1,189

Day 9
Breakfast: Mediterranean Frittata

Macro nutrition information

Carbohydrates— 8 grams

Fat— 5 grams

Protein— 11 grams

Kcal— 246

Lunch: Charcuterie Bistro Lunch

Macro nutrition information

Carbohydrates— 65 grams

Fat— 18 grams

Protein— 17 grams

Kcal— 452

Dinner: Italian Pasta Salad

Macro nutrition information

Carbohydrates— 42 grams

Fat— 20.1 grams

Protein— 17.2 grams

Kcal— 413

Total kcal for the day— 1, 111

Breakfast: Repeat meal from day 3

Macro nutrition information

Carbohydrates— 15 grams

Fat— 13 grams

Protein— 4 grams

Kcal— 306

Lunch: Mediterranean wrap

Macro nutrition information

Carbohydrates— 55 grams

Fat— 18 grams

Protein— 32 grams

Kcal— 501

Dinner: Tuna Salad

Macro nutrition information

Carbohydrates— 4.5 grams

Fat— 13.6 grams

Protein— 21.4 grams

Kcal— 225

Total kcal for the day— 1,032

Breakfast: Banana Nut Oatmeal

Macro nutrition information

Carbohydrates— 101.7 grams

Fat— 13.1 grams

Protein— 11.2 grams

Kcal— 532

Lunch: Mediterranean Kale and Lentil Salad

Macro nutrition information

Carbohydrates— 18 grams

Fat— 9 grams

Protein— 10 grams

Kcal— 186

Dinner: Mediterranean Pita sandwich

Macro nutrition information

Carbohydrates— 23.4 grams

Fat— 3 grams

Protein— 7.9 grams

Kcal— 147

Total kcal for the day— 865

Day 12

Breakfast: Garden-Fresh Omelets

Macro nutrition information

Carbohydrates— 9 grams

Fat— 12 grams

Protein— 15 grams

Kcal— 201

Lunch: Repeat meal from day 5

Macro nutrition information

Carbohydrates— 8 grams

Fat— 19 grams

Protein— 2 grams

Kcal— 198

Dinner: Italian Pasta Salad

Macro nutrition information

Carbohydrates— 42 grams

Fat— 20.1 grams

Protein— 17.2 grams

Kcal— 413

Total kcal for the day—812

Day 13
Breakfast: Banana Nut Oatmeal

Macro nutrition information

Carbohydrates— 101.7 grams

Fat— 13.1 grams

Protein— 11.2 grams

Kcal— 532

Lunch: Vegetable and Ravioli Soup

Macro nutrition information

Carbohydrates— 33 grams

Fat— 8 grams

Protein— 11 grams

Kcal— 261

Dinner: Chickpea Sauté and Greek Yogurt

Macro nutrition information

Carbohydrates— 28.4 grams

Fat— 25.3 grams

Protein— 10.5 grams

Kcal— 368

Total kcal for the day—1,161

Breakfast: Repeat meal from day 9

Macro nutrition information

Carbohydrates— 8 grams

Fat— 5 grams

Protein— 11 grams

Kcal— 246

Lunch: Cucumber Tomato White-Bean and Basil Vinaigrette Salad

Macro nutrition information

Carbohydrates— 22 grams

Fat— 15 grams

Protein— 8 grams

Kcal— 246

Dinner: Basil Garlic Shrimp Farrotto

Macro nutrition information

Carbohydrates— 46.2 grams

Fat— 13.7 grams

Protein— 27.2 grams

Kcal— 415

Total kcal for the day— 90

Chapter 8: Meal Prep and Planning

Meal Prepping and Its Benefits
Many people love to lead a healthy lifestyle, but first, you must ensure you are an organized individual. The truth is, it can get pretty difficult to stay organized when you have a busy schedule. Setting healthy goals for yourself can be easy but following through with them requires hard work and consistency.

As you already know, the Mediterranean diet consists of home cooked meals. Therefore, if you are going to start on this diet, it's important you follow it accordingly.

Remember, if you want to live a healthy lifestyle, you may have to make a few sacrifices. Once you get used to the routine, it will be easy. The whole concept of meal prepping deals with aspects of planning, arranging, packing, and organizing everything in advance. If you meal prep for a week, you will be able to manage your week's meal plan successfully. I'll be providing you with some tips and tricks to meal prepping. You don't necessarily have to stick to my method because meal prepping differs with each individual. You can use these tips and tricks to understand and create your own meal prep plan. Regardless of the format you follow, the meal prepping process should save you time and money. If you don't like to organize your meal prep for a whole week, you can do it only for a day.

Ultimately, its purpose is to help you save time, money, and energy.

It's best to understand some of the benefits related to meal prepping so that you will be motivated to follow it. So, let us discuss some of the benefits:

- You can save money by meal prepping. You should step away from the idea that healthy eating is costly, because it is not! If you plan your week's meals ahead, you will save money that would otherwise be spent on things you don't need. Buy items in bulk because you will be saving money when you do so. Planning ahead will aid you in purchasing only the things that are essential.

- You will witness positive changes in your weight. When you pre-plan, your time and effort is spent thinking about the ingredients you need and the recipes you will be making food from. Therefore, you also focus on the calories of each meal. This way, you are already unconsciously controlling your weight, because you are aware of the calories in each meal and the types of ingredients that are included.

- Prepare a list of things you need beforehand. This way, you won't stress yourself out over what you need and don't need. If you have a grocery shopping list, you will be able to control your spending and save time. I've added a shopping list at the end of this chapter for you so that you can get a brief understanding of what it should look like.

- You will be considerate about portion control, which is essential for weight loss. You will learn to balance your portions. You will not reach for more food than the food you already have stored in your cabinets.

Of course, you can treat yourself every now and then and indulge in more than you need to, but it's also important you manage your portions.

- You can control food waste. If you normally feel bad about throwing away food because it is spoiled or you couldn't finish it, meal prepping will save you from having to throw away your food. If you plan accordingly, you will not have leftovers and therefore, you won't have to throw away any food.

- Your overall health will benefit from meal planning. As you are meal prepping, you are aware of what you are going to eat. Therefore, you limit your less healthy options, and focus on the healthy ones instead. If you don't plan ahead, it's possible you will consume more unhealthy foods than healthy ones. Meal prepping allows you to plan your meals ahead.

- You will become a healthy version of yourself. Yes, willpower can be easily enhanced through healthy eating because with time, you will overcome cravings for unhealthy foods. If you are consistent, you will be able to avoid eating unhealthy foods without much effort.

- You will be stress-free. You will no longer need to stress about what you need to make for dinner, or what kind of snacks you can have in between meals. Eliminating stress will enhance your immune system and improve your sleep.

This list is just to be used as a general guideline. You will go through a period of trial and error until you find the right type of meal plan that works best for you. Once you become familiar with your plan, and remain consistent, you will meal prep effortlessly!

Meal Prep Tips and Ways to Save Money and Time
There are so many tips about meal prepping, but I have shortlisted a few important ones.

- Have everything that you need: You can't meal prep if you don't have the required utensils and ingredients. Before you start meal prepping, you must get your week's meal plan ingredients along with the needed appliances. Don't overlook items like a sharp knife and measuring cup when you are meal prepping because you need them. You should have them ready when you begin meal prepping.

- Meal plan: This is one of the most important tips because it helps you stay organized. The meal plan will give a clear idea of what to do next!

- Get the required containers: Without containers, you will not be able to meal prep, so purchase them beforehand and keep them near you. There are different styles of containers that you can get for reasonable prices.

- Double batch meals: There are certain meals that you can double batch and freeze. For example, you can do this with casseroles. So, when you are prepping, make sure to increase the measurements. If you do so, you will be able to manage busy nights without dumping junk into your stomach. Also, it will save you money when you purchase ingredients in bulk.

- Cook dinner early: If you can wake up early and prepare dinner along with breakfast, you're ahead of the game. Or, if you can cook dinner during lunch, you will also save more time. Also, if prep everything beforehand, cooking will not be a big deal.

- Keep snacks ready: You don't have to stress about preparing snacks every morning. Instead, you can prepare snacks for a week and store them away for when you want them. Some ideas for snacks include a muffin with some fruit or Greek yogurt with strawberries. There are many simple snack recipes that you can prepare effortlessly.

- Shop during the right season: If you can shop during the right season for certain fruits and vegetables, you will be able to get cheaper, and great quality fruits and vegetables.

- Purchase staple items in bulk: Buy items like spices and herbs in bulk, since you'll be using them in almost all your recipes anyway. Not only will you save time, but you will also be saving money if you do this.

Follow these meal prep tips and make meal prepping fun!

How to Meal Plan and What Makes a Healthy Meal Plan?

What does the word 'healthy' mean? Most people assume healthy means sacrificing taste and preferences. However, when following the Mediterranean diet, you don't have to sacrifice taste, experience, or preference. A healthy meal plan begins at home. What does this mean? This means that you put in the time and effort to prepare your meals at home. Do not resort to eating junk food or fast food that you can buy on the go. A healthy meal plan consists of a plan and list of recipes that can be cooked right at home.

When you prepare food at home, you know exactly what ingredients will be going into your food. But when you buy food outside of home, you don't know what ingredients people have put into that food, therefore it is impossible to label it is as 'healthy,' even if you think it might be. If you know the food ingredients, calorie count, nutrition count, and everything else, you will be able to decide whether it can be considered healthy or not. The meals you eat should make you feel satiated and nourished, and that's what defines healthy eating.

A healthy eating plan can be created easily when you follow the Mediterranean diet as the diet itself makes everything clear for you!

How to Store and Freeze Your Meals, Food Safety, and Re-Heating Your Meals?

You can't fit all the foods in the fridge because some need a different method of storing. The foods that are kept in the fridge are stored that way to slow down the growth of germs and to keep them fresh. If you look at the labels on the packaging of milk, meat, and fish, you will find the "keep refrigerated" mark on it. If you happen to purchase canned foods, you should not refrigerate them because the metal from the can will seep into the food. You should also follow the storage instructions on the can's label accordingly.

When freezing meals, make sure to store them in an airtight container. Freezer bags are a good option as well.

Also, remember you can freeze almost all the types of foods. When you are storing poultry, you have to really be careful so as not to cause any bacterial growth on the poultry. If you store the poultry in the fridge, you will avoid both bacterial growth and food poisoning. If you have cooked poultry, keep it separate from the raw poultry.

What about defrosting fish and meat? If you are planning to eat meat occasionally, it is essential to know its storage methods. You can freeze both fish and meat for a long time (but better to not keep it frozen for too long). Before cooking the meat or fish that you froze, it is important you defrost completely.

When you are defrosting meat or fish, you must get rid of the excess liquid neatly and carefully without letting it spread everywhere. If you are planning on cooking it right away, you can use the microwave to defrost it faster. Remember, after defrosting it, you have to consume it within a day. After defrosting food, you shouldn't reheat the food twice. There is a greater chance of bacteria developing if you continuously freeze the food after it's been defrosted.

You have to be cautious when dealing with foods that need to be stored, defrosted, or reheated. You shouldn't be careless about storing food because even the slightest mistake can lead to more significant issues. Be responsible when you are storing food!

Grocery Shopping List
Staples

- Olive oil
- Extra-virgin olive oil
- Balsamic vinegar
- Parsley Oregano
- Cinnamon
- Basil
- Cumin
- Pepper
- Cloves

- Coriander
- Fennel seeds
- Dill
- Rosemary
- Ginger
- Garlic
- Tahini
- Hummus
- Canned and packaged
- Olive
- Whole grain bread

Pantry

- Whole grain pasta
- Legumes
- White beans
- Chickpeas
- Black beans
- Red kidney beans
- Buckwheat
- Brown rice
- Whole-wheat couscous
- Barley

- Quinoa
- Faro
- Oats
- Almonds
- Hazelnuts
- Sesame seeds
- Cashews
- Walnuts
- Peanuts
- Pistachios
- Sunflower seeds

Produce

- Eggplants
- Onions
- Tomatoes
- Zucchinis
- Apples
- Mushrooms
- Oranges
- Pears
- Grapes
- Bananas

- Artichokes
- Avocado
- Asparagus
- Broccoli
- Dates
- Beets
- Brussels sprouts
- Carrots
- Cabbage
- Cucumbers
- Cherries
- Figs
- Limes
- Mushrooms
- Melons
- Squash
- Spinach
- Pomegranate

Fish and Meat

- Chicken
- Tuna
- Salmon

- Haddock
- Mackerel
- Turkey
- Mussels
- Shellfish
- Scallops
- Tilapia
- Clams
- Crab
- Red meat (in moderation)

Dairy and Eggs

- Greek yogurt
- Low-fat milk
- Eggs
- Goat cheese
- Parmesan
- Mozzarella

Meal Prep
Breakfast: Buckwheat and Chia Seed Porridge

This is a delicious breakfast option that is also rich in anti-inflammatory properties. The buckwheat grain has a good texture, is gluten free and a good substitute for oats. The chia seed topping gives this dish a fresh taste and the omega 3 minimizes inflammation and stops joint stiffness. This recipe also contains a lot of protein and fiber which will keep you feeling full for longer.

Total prep & cook time: 30 minutes

Serving yields: 5 servings

Nutritional facts: 320 calories/ 66g net carbs/ 3g total fats/ 12g protein

Ingredients needed: Chia Seeds 2 tablespoons, Water 2 cups, Apple (1, grated, with skin on), Pear (1, grated, with skin on), Oats 0.5 cups, Buckwheat 1 cup (rinsed), a pinch of Ginger, Cinnamon, Cardamom and Nutmeg each, Nut butter 2 tablespoons, Vanilla Extract 1 teaspoon, and Honey 2 tablespoons.

Directions

1. Put 1 cup of milk in a bowl and add the chia seeds.
2. Put 1 cup of water in another bowl and add the buckwheat and oats
3. Leave both bowls to soak overnight
4. In the morning, drain water from both buckwheat and oats, rinsing them thoroughly
5. Place a medium saucepan over medium heat
6. Place the chia seeds with the milk into the saucepan. Add the remaining milk (1 cup). Also add the other ingredients (nut butter, grated apple and pear, vanilla, honey, buckwheat, oats, and all of the spices)
7. Simmer and cook for 18 minutes, constantly stirring to achieve a thick and creamy porridge. As you stir, add more water to achieve the consistency you want.
8. Serve the porridge in cups

Additional tip: This porridge can stay in the refrigerator for up to 5 days. You can cook a lot and then warm each serving as taken

Lunch: Avocado Sandwich with Grilled Sauerkraut

This meal contains anti-inflammatory properties equivalent to those found in the anti-inflammatory drug Reuben. Since it has less calories and salt than Reuben, it is less likely to cause weight gain. One of its most crucial ingredients, Sauerkraut, has probiotics that suppress inflammatory arthritis inside the intestine's walls.

Total prep & cook time: 22 minutes

Serving yields: 4

Nutritional facts: 319 calories/ 39 net carbs/ 14g total fats/ 10g protein

Ingredients needed: Pumpernickel Bread 8 slices, Vegan Butter, Hummus 1 cup (roasted garlic flavor), Sauerkraut (rinsed and drained), avocado 1 (peeled and cut into slices)

Directions:

1. Butter all slices of bread and arrange them on a baking sheet
2. Distribute 0.5 cup hummus on 4 slices of bread

3. Add sauerkraut on top of the hummus on each slice
4. Place avocado slices on top of the sauerkraut and hummus
5. Distribute hummus on the other 4 slices and place them over the avocados
6. Place in the oven heated to 180 degrees Celsius for 8 minutes, then change the sides and cook for up to 6 more minutes.
7. The sandwiches are ready when crunchy and golden brown.

Dinner: Salmon with Zucchini Pesto and Pasta

This recipe is a simple meal with plenty of omega-3 fatty acids. Zucchini pasta is the perfect substitution for pasta. Also, Salmon can be a smart substitute for deep sea fatty fish such as mackerel or tuna.

Total prep & cook time: 25 minutes

Serving yields: 4

Nutritional facts: 236 calories/ 11.2 net carbs/ 10.3g total fats/ 25.7g protein

Ingredients needed: Zucchini 1 medium or large, Avocado 1, Parmesan 0.25 cup grated, Lemon 1, Black Pepper up to 1 tablespoon depending on how you like black pepper, and Salmon steaks 2 defrosted.

Directions:

1. Season the salmon steaks with black pepper and lemon juice and place them on a baking sheet
2. Place the steaks in the oven for 18 minutes over 180 degrees Celsius
3. Cut the zucchini into thin slices or noodles
4. Mash avocado in a bowl, add pesto, pepper and the remaining lemon juice.
5. Once the salmon is cooked, serve it on plates adding the zucchini slices and the mashed avocado.

Additional tip: You can leave the avocado ingredient out of this recipe to lower fat content.

Breakfast: Oat Porridge with Berries

This recipe contains numerous fibers, antioxidants and probiotics, all helpful for anti-inflammation. Oats are high in fiber and a rich source of Bifidobacterium bacteria, necessary for preventing diabetes related to inflammation. Berries are good antioxidants and produce an anti-inflammatory element known as anthocyanins.

Total prep & cook time: 30

Serving yields: 4

Nutritional facts: 68 calories/ 12g net carbs/ 1.4g total fats/ 2.4g protein

Ingredients needed: Steel cut oats 1 cup, Water 3 cups, Salt a pinch, and fresh Berries (both blueberries or raspberries can work).

Directions:

1. Heat a large sized saucepan and add the oats
2. Cook for about 3 minutes, stirring frequently to allow cohesive toasting
3. Add the 3 cups of water and once it begins to boil, simmer for about 18 minutes to cook the oats
4. Additional tip: You can try using other sweeteners such as few drops of stevia, hemp seeds or kefir. Also, if you prefer the end product thicker, add some milk while the oats cook.

This recipe is a simple delicacy that contains anti-inflammatory elements in large quantities. Spinach is a leafy green so has high levels of polyphenols, which suppress inflammatory conditions such as diabetes and multiple sclerosis.

Total prep & cook time: 20 minutes

Serving yields: 4

Nutritional facts: 153 calories/ 11.5g net carbs/ 5.6g total fats/ 1.2g protein

Ingredients needed: olive oil 1 teaspoon, brown onion small, peeled and chopped finely, baby spinach 0.25 kg, eggs 4, feta cheese 0.5 cup and crumbled, salt and black pepper 0.5 teaspoon each, and garlic 1 teaspoon.

Directions:

1. Heat the olive oil using a non-stick medium sized pan in the oven. Once hot, add onions and cook for 3 minutes.

2. Add spinach while stirring gently for 2 to 3 minutes until the leaves shrivel. Set it aside.
3. Put the 4 eggs in a dish. Add the spinach, feta, and seasonings (black pepper and salt).
4. Heat the pan again and add the egg mixture. Cook for about 10 minutes, stirring gently until the egg settles at the bottom
5. Turn off the heat but leave the pan on the grill until the frittata is cooked to golden brown (about 2-3 minutes).
6. Serve hot or cold

Additional tip: Side salads can be added to benefit the meal and the body.

Dinner: Sweet Potato with Lentil and Chicken Soup

This recipe is delicious and contains fiber, proteins and vitamins necessary for anti-inflammation. Sweet potatoes have vitamins, nutrients and helpful antioxidants. The lentil soup option improves the fiber and protein content of this meal.

Total prep & cook time: 30 minutes

Serving yields: 5

Nutritional facts: 529 calories/ 34g net carbs/ 31g total fats/ 28g protein

Ingredients needed: Chicken carcass 1, cooked and shredded chicken 0.5 cups, sweet potatoes 2 chopped into small pieces, salt 1 teaspoon, virgin olive oil 2 tablespoons, water 8 cups, celery stalks 10 and sliced into 0.5 inch pieces, garlic cloves 6 and noodle-thin sliced, head escarole 0.5 cups, chopped into small pieces, lentils 0.75 cups and well rinsed, and lemon 1.

Directions:

1. Pour water in a medium sized pot. Add potatoes, chicken carcass, lentils and salt.
2. Place the pot on stove top over high heat and bring to a boil. Simmer for about 10 minutes until sweet potatoes become tender.
3. Set the pot aside and remove the chicken carcass.
4. Put a pot over medium high heat and add oil. Add celery and garlic and cook for 7 minutes.

5. Add shredded chicken and escarole, and simmer. Add salt and wait for about 3 minutes to ensure that the escarole has softened.
6. Add lemon juice to the pot. It is now ready to serve.

Breakfast: Buckwheat Pancakes and Berries

Buckwheat is a remarkable ingredient for anti-inflammatory breakfast menus. The good thing about it is that it is available in most grocery stores and can be shopped online. It is rich in anti-inflammatory components, like rutin and quercetin. These are good antioxidants that can help in suppressing arthritis associated with inflammation. Best of all, buckwheat is also gluten free. This meal is easy and quick to prepare and has an incredible flavor.

Total prep & cook time: 25 minutes

Serving yields: 8

Nutritional facts: 144 calories/ 19.42g net carbs/ 5.1g total fats/ 5.42g protein

Ingredients needed: Buckwheat flour 1.5 cups, sugar 4 teaspoons, baking soda 2 pinches, buttermilk 1.25 cups, egg 1 large, a pinch of vanilla extract, a pinch of salt, Butter 2 teaspoons, strawberries 1 pint chopped into halves.

Directions:

1. Mix the dry batter ingredients in a large dish
2. Add egg and vanilla extract into another bowl and add milk. Stir until even.
3. Add the milk, egg and vanilla concoction into the dry ingredients bowl and combine to obtain a good texture.
4. Measure batter using a 0.5 cup level and place each measure on a warm pan.
5. Allow it to cook for about a minute or two until there are small bubbles on the pancakes' surface.
6. Turn sides to allow pancake to cook.
7. You will know it is ready when it's golden brown on both sides. Repeat the process for the rest of the batter.

8. Put the pancakes in the oven and wait for 2 minutes. Serve the pancakes when hot and serve it with the strawberries.

Additional tip: You can use other berries such as blueberries or raspberries.

Lunch: Citrus Salad and Quinoa

This is a quick and easy recipe to prepare and it qualifies as a vegan anti-inflammatory diet option. The citrus fruit gives the meal a touch of antioxidants and the vitamin C helps the body absorb iron from quinoa.

Total prep & cook time: 20 minutes

Serving yields: 1

Nutritional facts: 111 calories/ 0.4g net carbs/ 5.0g total fats/ 1.8g protein

Ingredients needed: Cooked and cooled Quinoa 1 cup, celery rib 1 sliced finely, onion 1 green and chopped, fresh parsley 0.5 cup chopped, and oranges 2 small.

Dressing ingredients needed: 2 drops of lemon juice, white wine vinegar 0.5 tablespoons, juice from one of the oranges, salt 0.5 teaspoons, a small pinch of black pepper, 0.5 teaspoons of cinnamon, and fresh ginger 0.5 teaspoons grated.

Directions:

1. Cut one orange into 4 pieces and squeeze out the juice from the orange pieces into a bowl.
2. Put the juice in a blender and add all of the dressing ingredients to the blender.
3. Blend until a smooth texture is achieved.
4. Chop the other orange pieces into bite sized pieces and add the remaining ingredients. Stir until even.
5. Serve immediately or preserve in the refrigerator.

Additional tip: This meal stays fresh when refrigerated; it can be prepared in advance, stored and retrieved later. Also, the ingredients can be doubled or tripled for more servings.

Dinner: Cauliflower Rice and Salmon with Greens

This recipe is highly nutritious and contains anti-inflammatory properties. It is an easy meal for the evening. Cauliflower rice is a substitute for regular rice, for the direct purpose of anti-inflammation. Both cauliflower and salmon are rich in polyphenols, fiber and antioxidants.

Total prep & cook time: 30 mins

Serving yields: 2

Nutritional facts: 261 calories/ 7.1g net carbs/ 2.1g total fats/ 4.5g protein

Ingredients needed: Brussels sprouts 12 sliced into halves, roasted and cooled, Kale 1 bunch rinsed and cut into small pieces, cauliflower 0.5 head beaten into cauliflower rice, a pinch of salt, olive or coconut oil 0.25 cups, and organic salmon 2 units.

Marinade ingredients needed: tamari sauce 0.25 cups, sesame oil 0.5 tablespoons, honey 1 teaspoon, and dijon mustard 1 teaspoon.

Directions:

1. Thoroughly combine all marinade ingredients in a dish.
2. Put the roasted brussel sprouts halves on a baking tray.
3. Add Salmon fillets on top.
4. Distribute marinade over the fillets and put in the oven to cook for about 15 minutes.
5. Heat the olive/coconut oil in a large pan.
6. Sauté the kale for up to 3 minutes for them to wilt. Remove from the pan.
7. Heat 1 tablespoon oil in pan and add cauliflower rice. Add a pinch of salt, curry powder and sauté for up to 3 minutes
8. Serve.

Additional tip: If cauliflower is not your thing, you can mix it with brown rice to add more taste. Also, a whole cauliflower could be used based if you do like it.

Breakfast: Ginger Muffins with Apple and Rhubarb

A good meal to begin your day with, easy to make and anti-inflammatory. Rhubarb helps in curbing the formation of inflammatory diseases. It prevents inflammation related diseases such as rheumatoid arthritis and appendicitis. Ginger helps to ease arthritis pain and it also offers a great taste.

Total prep & cook time: 30

Serving yields: 8

Nutritional facts: 196g calories/ 5.1g net carbs/ 4.1g total fats/ 6.2g protein

Ingredients needed: Crystalized ginger 2 tablespoons, organic corn flour 2 tablespoons, baking powder 2 tablespoons, cinnamon 0.5 teaspoon, ginger 0.5 teaspoon, salt 0.5 teaspoon, almond meal 0.5 cups, buckwheat flour 0.5 cups, brown rice flour 0.5 cups, ground linseed meal 1 tablespoon, brown sugar 0.25 cup, Apple 1 small and finely chopped, rhubarb 1 cup finely chopped, vanilla extract 1 teaspoon, egg 1 medium, olive oil 2 tablespoons, almond milk 0.75 cup.

Directions:

1. Line 8 muffin tins with paper liners or grease each tin.

2. Combine sugar, ginger, almond meal, and linseed meal in a medium sized bowl.

3. Add baking powder, flours, and spices to the bowl. Mix all ingredients thoroughly.

4. Add apple and rhubarb to the flour mixture

5. In another medium sized bowl, beat the egg, adding the vanilla and milk. Combine and add to the flour mixture. Mix thoroughly.

6. Divide the batter in to the 8 muffin tins.

7. Bake for approximately 20 minutes. You know they are ready once golden and well risen. You can test with a small knife. (If the knife comes out clean, they're ready.

8. Set them aside on a wire rack to allow them cool further.They are ready to eat

Additional tip: They can be eaten when prepared, and they can also stay fresh for up to 3 days if stored in airtight containers.

Lunch: Tuna Salad

This is an easy med-diet recipe and a great source of n-3 fatty acids. It is delicious when served with greens or spread over whole grain bread, all of which are anti-inflammatory.

Total prep & cook time: 25 minutes

Serving yields: 4

Nutritional facts: 187g calories/ 9g net carbs/ 9g total fats/ 16g protein

Ingredients needed: mayonnaise 0.25 cup, olives 0.25 cup, red onion 1 chopped, tuna 2 cans drained, roasted red peppers 2 tablespoons, capers 1 tablespoon, and ripe tomatoes 2 large.

Directions:

1. In a large bowl, mix all the ingredients except the tomatoes.
2. Cut both tomatoes 6 times without separating the pieces.
3. Open the tomatoes gently and scoop the tuna salad into the tomatoes. Serve

Additional tip: I recommend choosing canned tuna that is low sodium.

Dinner: Tilapia with Rosemary Topping

This is an easy and quick fix anti-inflammatory recipe. It has various anti-inflammatory properties such as selenium from the tilapia and antioxidants in the rosemary. Selenium helps to suppress inflammation related arthritis.

Total prep & cook time: 30 minutes

Serving yields: 5

Nutritional facts: 222 calories/ 6.7 g net carbs/ 10.8 g total fats/ 26.8g protein

Ingredients needed: Raw pecans 1 cup chopped, whole wheat panko breadcrumbs 1 cup, fresh rosemary 2 teaspoons, brown or coconut palm sugar 1 teaspoon, a pinch of cayenne pepper, 2 pinches of salt, olive oil 1.5 teaspoon, egg white 1, and tilapia fillets 4.

Directions:

1. Heat the oven to 350 degrees Fahrenheit.
2. Beat the egg in a shallow dish. Add olive oil and stir

3. In a medium sized bowl mix the breadcrumbs, rosemary, sugar, pecans, pepper and salt.
4. Taking one tilapia at a time, dip them in the eggs and then in the breadcrumb mixture, covering fully, and place each one on a non-stick pan.
5. Distribute any residual breadcrumb concoction on top of the fish and bake for 7 minutes. Food is ready to serve.

Breakfast: Crepes

Crepes are one of the best and easiest breakfast meals. Light and tasty, they are anti-inflammatory and gluten-free pancakes.

Total prep & cook time: 30 minutes

Serving yields: 6

Nutritional facts: 90 calories/ 6g net carbs/ 5.2g total fats/ 4.6g protein

Ingredients needed: egg 1, nut milk 0.5 cup, water 0.5 cup, a pinch of salt, agave nectar 1 tablespoon, wheat flour 1 cup, vanilla 1 teaspoon, coconut oil 3 tablespoons.

Directions:

1. Melt coconut oil in a pan over medium heat
2. Mix the milk, salt, water, vanilla, eggs and nectar in a dish.
3. Add flour and combine
4. Measure scoops of about 0.25 cups of batter on the pan at a time. Swirl the pan in a slow motion to spread batter. Leave it for 1.5 minutes to cook. Flip the sides to allow all parts to cook. You will know it is ready once golden brown all over.
5. Repeat the process for the remaining batter

Additional tip: They are best served with berries, either blueberries or raspberries.

Lunch: Salmon Potato Tartine with Salad

This dish is a great anti-inflammatory lunch option. Salmon is rich in omega 3 and the salad greens are rich in antioxidants.

Total prep & cook time: 28 minutes

Serving yields: 4

Nutritional facts: 337g calories/ 4.8g net carbs/ 16.5g total fats/ 2.5g protein

Ingredients needed: Potato 1 large peeled and cut lengthways, salt 0.5 teaspoon, a pinch of black pepper, butter 2 tablespoons, soft goat cheese 4 oz., chopped chives 3 teaspoons, garlic cloves 0.5, salmon smoked and thinly cut, boiled egg half, minced chives for garnish, lemon 0.5, zest of half a lemon, and garlic clove 0.5 finely chopped

Directions:

1. Combine goat cheese, lemon and garlic in a dish. Add pepper and salt to season. Set aside
2. Add salt to the onion and boiled egg to season
3. Grate the potato using the large grating holes. Drain any excess liquid from the potato. Add a pinch of salt and pepper to season
4. Using a non-stick large pan, heat the butter. Put the grated potato in the pan when the butter is hot.
5. Make the mixture compact and solid with the spatula, leave it for up to 7 minutes until golden brown at the bottom

6. Flip and cook the other side for up to 6 minutes until golden brown

7. Remove and cool for about 5 minutes. Once cooled, distribute the goat cheese mixture on top, then salmon, onions, egg and capers. Finally, add the sliced chives.

8. Cut into desired shapes and serve.

Dinner: Potato Curry and Poached Eggs

Eggs are a good source of omega 3 fatty acids, especially those directly purchased from the farm. Also, potatoes contain anti-inflammatory components such as anthocyanin, and resistant starch. This is an easy meal for lunch or dinner and quick to prepare.

Total prep & cook time: 30 minutes

Serving yields: 4

Nutritional facts: 156 calories/ 20g net carbs/ 1g total fats/ 1g protein

Ingredients needed: Russet potatoes 2, ginger 1 inch, garlic 2 cloves, olive oil 2 teaspoons, eggs 4 large, curry powder 2 tablespoons, cilantro 0.5 bunch.

Directions:

1. Cut peeled potatoes into bite sizes. Add them in a pot of water over high heat. Cover and let them boil for 4 minutes. Remove water and leave the potatoes to cool.
2. Grate ginger into a large sized pot.
3. Add the olive oil, ginger and garlic. Heat the pot for about 3 minutes.
4. Add curry powder and wait for another minute before adding the tomato sauce. Add a pinch of salt to season.
5. Put the cooled potatoes into the pot and cover them with the sauce. If the mixture feels dry, add ¼ cup of water.
6. Using a spatula, create 4 dips in the mixture and insert an egg into each.
7. Cover and simmer for up to 8 minutes.
8. Food is ready. Serve with coriander or fresh parsley.

Breakfast: Vegetable Curry with Brown Rice

Veggies are a good source of anti-inflammatory properties such as antioxidants. Brown rice is a good substitute for oatmeal or whole wheat bread and is high in fiber. This is an easy Thai-inspired meal to make and an all-time delicacy.

Total prep & cook time: 26 minutes

Serving yields: 4

Nutritional facts: 665 calories/ 80g net carbs/ 31 g total fats/ 26g protein

Ingredients needed: Red onion 1 chopped, olive oil 1 tablespoon, bell pepper 1, fresh ginger sliced 1 tablespoon, garlic cloves 3 ground, small head cauliflower 1 cut into small pieces, chili powder 2 teaspoons, finely ground coriander 1 teaspoon, red curry paste 3 tablespoons, coconut milk 14 oz. tin, peas 2 cups, a pinch of salt, a pinch of black pepper, steamed brown rice, fresh coriander leaves 0.25 cup, scallions 4 and thinly sliced, and cooked chickpeas 28 oz. tin.

Directions:

1. Using a medium sized frypan, heat oil.
2. Cook onions and peppers in the pan
3. Add ginger and garlic to season and simmer for three minutes
4. Add the cauliflower after 3 minutes. Use a spatula to stir and ensure it is well combined.
5. Add the coriander, red curry and chili powder. Wait for the mixture to darken slightly, about one minute.
6. Add milk into the pot and allow to simmer. Wait for the cauliflower to become soft.
7. Add lime juice into the pot and ensure it is well combined.
8. Add peas and chickpeas. Add pepper and salt to season. Simmer for 2-3 minutes.
9. Food is ready. Serve with rice. Top up with scallions and coriander.

Poke is a fatty fish with a high level of omega 3 fatty acid content. The ginger vinaigrette is made with anti-inflammatory ingredient such as garlic and ginger. Also, this meal is easy and quick to prepare.

Total prep & cook time: 25 minutes

Serving yields: 4

Nutritional facts: 730 calories/ net carbs/ total fats/ protein

Ingredients needed:

Tuna poke ingredients: toasted sesame seeds 2 tablespoons, honey 0.25 cup, garlic sauce 1 teaspoon, corn starch 1 teaspoon, pineapple juice 0.25 cup, tuna steaks 2, wonton wrappers and soy sauce 10 mls.

For the vinaigrette: soy sauce 10 mls, hot chili sesame oil 0.5 cup, tahini 1 tablespoon, freshly grounded ginger 2 teaspoons, ground garlic 0.5 clove, sesame seeds 1 tablespoon, and pineapple and vinegar liquids 0.25 cup each

Salad ingredients: red chili 1 chopped, fresh pineapple sliced 1 cup, avocado, fresh coriander 0.5 cup, and spring greens 1 cup.

Directions:

1. Grease a baking sheet and lay the wonton strips. Spray olive oil on the wontons and season with a pinch of salt.
2. Bake for up to 8 minutes in a high heat oven. They are cooked when crispy and golden brown. Set aside to cool.
3. Make the sauce by mixing soy sauce, cornstarch, honey, and pineapple juice, together with garlic sauce in a large cooking pot.
4. Heat the pot on the stove and bring to a boil. Allow the sauce to simmer, waiting for approximately 3 minutes as the sauce begins to thicken. It is ready if it sticks on the spoon. Remove the pot from heat and set aside

5. Heat sesame oil in another pot, a large one preferably.

6. Add in the fish and cook for 3 minutes before flipping, searing both sides evenly. Once complete, about 2 minutes, remove the steaks from the heat.

7. Brush either side of the steaks with the soy sauce mixture prepared before. Chop the steak into strips.

8. In a separate bowl, combine coriander, pineapple pieces, red chili, avocado, and spring greens. Stir to combine.

9. In a separate dish, mix the remaining soy sauce, pineapple juice, hot chili, sesame oil, garlic sauce, rice vinegar, lime, lime zest, and sesame seeds to make the vinaigrette. Season with some fresh garlic and ginger.

10. Food is ready. Serve the greens with the steak and sauce mixtures layered.

11. Garnish with avocado slices, tuna and wonton crisps on top. Sprinkle with vinaigrette.

Dinner: Chicken Coated with Balsamic Vinegar, Pumpkin Seeds, Cranberries and Broccoli

This is a juicy meal that is easy and quick to make. Broccoli is one of the most remarkable cruciferous vegetables and has a great anti-inflammatory potency. Broccoli is also yummy. The balsamic vinegar helps to keep chicken juicy.

Total prep & cook time: 20

Serving yields: 4

Nutritional facts: 1857 calories/ 114g net carbs/ 69g total fats/ 195g protein

Ingredients needed: balsamic vinegar 0.25 cup, honey 2 tablespoons, olive oil 3 tablespoons, broccoli 2 cups, chicken breast 1.25 pounds cut into pieces, black pepper and salt each a pinch, shallot 1 large and chopped into pieces, cranberries 0.5 cup, dry tomatoes 0.5 cup, roasted pumpkin seeds 0.5 cup.

Directions:

1. Using a large cooking pan, heat 2 tablespoons of olive oil, add the broccoli pieces and allow to cook for approximately 3 minutes.
2. Flip the broccoli over to cook on all sides. You know they are ready when they are bright and el dante.
3. Pile the broccoli onto one side of the pan and put the remaining olive oil on the empty side. Add in the chicken and shallots. Cook for up to 4 minutes while stirring and gently flipping sides.
4. Sprinkle balsamic vinegar over the chicken, add in honey and stir gently.
5. Simmer for 4 minutes to allow the chicken to cook fully. By now the broccoli will be quite tender.
6. Distribute sun-dried tomatoes, pumpkin seeds, cranberries, and combine gently.
7. Serve while still hot.

Additional tip: Meal is best enjoyed on the day of cooking but can stay fresh for some time in the refrigerator.

Breakfast: Flat Bread and Ricotta Artichoke

This meal is rich in anti-inflammatory properties and it is also a delicacy to start your day with. Artichoke is a dark veggie and it is rich in anti-inflammatory oxidants. Flat bread is a whole-food which boosts anti-oxidation, thus reducing inflammation. Ricotta is rich in n-3 fatty acids. On top of that, this meal is speedy and stress-free to make.

Total prep & cook time: 20 minutes

Serving yields: 4

Nutritional facts: 551 calories/ 9g net carbs/ 8.9g total fats/ 2.3g protein

Ingredients needed: olive oil 2 teaspoons, honey 1 tablespoon, artichokes 8 oz. marinated and dried, arugula 3 cups, chives 1 tablespoon chopped, whole milk ricotta cheese 2 cups, pizza dough 0.5 pounds, basil 2 tablespoons chopped, mozzarella 6 oz., fresh shaved parmesan cheese 0.5 cup.

Vinaigrette ingredients: a pinch of salt, apple cider vinegar 1 tablespoon, lemon 1, and olive oil 4 teaspoons.

Directions:

1. Prepare a large baking tray by greasing with olive oil.
2. Mold the dough into a thin piece by rolling it on a surface with flour. Put it on the baking tray and sprinkle it with olive oil on top. Season the dough to your liking.
3. Place the baking tray in the oven under a 450 degrees F heat. Bake for 10 minutes or until the dough becomes golden brown. Take the bread out of the oven and set aside to cool.
4. In a medium sized bowl combine basil, honey, ricotta, and a pinch of black pepper and salt.
5. Spread the ricotta on top of the bread. Add the artichokes on top. Top it with prosciutto and mozzarella. If you are feeling fancy, even distribute arugula and parmesan.
6. Sprinkle the topping with lemon vinaigrette and serve immediately.

Lunch: Pineapple Fried Brown Rice

Pineapple is simply delicious and a great fruit for anti-inflammatory purposes. It contains an element known as bromelain which aids in suppressing the inflammatory responses of the body. It adds a special taste to the brown rice, also known as a powerful anti-inflammatory food.

Total prep & cook time: 30 minutes

Serving yields: 4

Nutritional facts: 111 calories/ 23g net carbs/ 0.9g total fats/ 2.6g protein

Ingredients needed: corn and peas each 1 cup, pineapple 2 cups chopped into pieces, ham 0.5 cup chopped, green onions 2 chopped, 1 red onion chopped, carrots 2 grated, ground garlic 2 cloves, olive oil 2 tablespoons, a pinch of pepper, ginger powder 0.5 teaspoon, sesame oil 2 teaspoons, cooked brown rice 3 cups, and soy sauce 3 tablespoons.

Directions:

1. Mix together soy sauce, ginger powder, pepper, sesame oil and the ground ginger in a dish.
2. Heat the oil in a medium sized cooking pan. Add garlic and onions allow them to cook for about five minutes.
3. Add corn, carrots, and peas. Stir gently and constantly to ensure that the vegetables become tender, do this for about 5 minutes.
4. Add rice, ham, pineapple, green onions, pineapple and the sauce mixture prepared before to the pan. Stir constantly for 3 minutes to allow the contents to heat thoroughly. Serve while hot.

Dinner: Mackerel Baked in Sesame and Ginger, in Parchment

Mackerel is a delicious fatty fish and it has a lot of omega 3 fatty acids. This meal is packed with veggies and natural spices such as ginger and garlic, which are high in anti-inflammatory properties. It is also an easy meal to prepare and ideal for a quick dinner.

Total prep & cook time: 30

Serving yields: 4

Nutritional facts: 468 calories/ 21g net carbs/ 26g total fats/ 39g protein

Ingredients needed: lime 1 and cut into 4 pieces, zucchini 1 large and thinly chopped, red onion 1 and chopped, skinless mackerel fillets 4, sesame seeds 4 teaspoons, oil 1 teaspoon, soy sauce 2 tablespoons, ginger 2 tablespoons freshly grated, honey 2 tablespoons, garlic powder 1 teaspoon, and a pinch of black pepper.

Directions:

1. Prepare 4 parchment sections. Fold each piece twice to make a line and then unfold.
2. Mix garlic powder, soy sauce, black pepper and honey in a medium sized bowl and set aside
3. Back to the parchment sections, take one at a time and put a piece of the zucchini on one side of the line.
4. On top of the zucchini, place some red onions. Add lime from one the four pieces of the cut lime.

5. Put a mackerel fillet on top. Distribute the soy sauce mixture made before on top of the fillet. Add 1 teaspoon of sesame seeds.

6. Cover this content with the empty side of the parchment and fold the edges to seal the package fully.

7. Repeat this process with the remaining ingredients and parchments.

8. Put the parchment packs in the oven at a heat of 350 degrees Fahrenheit.

9. Let it cook for up to 18 minutes. Serve while hot.

Additional tip: You can serve by cutting the top of the parchment and serving the fish inside of the parchment sections, or you can remove the fish and veggies from the parchment sections and serve on plates.

Breakfast: Eggs, Tomatoes and Asparagus

Eggs contain omega-3 fatty acids, which help in anti-inflammation. This meal is quick to prepare and it is an energizing meal to start your day.

Total prep & cook time: 30 minutes

Serving yields: 4

Nutritional facts: 158 calories/ 13g net carbs/ 11g total fats/ 11g protein

Ingredients needed: 4 eggs, olive oil 2 tablespoons, thyme 2 teaspoons, a pinch of salt and pepper, asparagus 2 pounds and cherry tomatoes 1 pint.

Directions:

1. Prepare a baking sheet
2. Place the cherry tomatoes and asparagus on the baking sheet. Sprinkle olive oil and use salt, pepper and thyme to season.
3. Place the baking sheet inside the oven at 400 degrees fahrenheit for 12 minutes or until the contents are golden.
4. Remove from heat and add the eggs on top of the baking sheet contents, then return it to the oven and cook for up to 8 minutes.
5. Serve when hot.

Lunch: Mediterranean Baked Sweet Potatoes

Sweet potatoes are a sweet meal and a good source of anti-inflammatory nutrients. They contain a lot of vitamin E and C as well as the carotenoid beta carotene, all of which reduces inflammation.

Total prep & cook time: 30

Serving yields: 4

Nutritional facts: 313 calories/ 60g net carbs/ 5g total fats/ 8.6g protein

Ingredients needed: chickpeas 100 ounce can, sweet potatoes 4 medium, olive oil 1 teaspoon, salt 0.25 teaspoon, coriander, cumin, paprika and cinnamon each 0.5 teaspoon.

Garlic herb sauce: Water 0.5 cup, a pinch of sea salt, ground garlic 3 cloves, dried dill 1 teaspoon, lemon 0.5, and hummus 0.25 cup.

Toppings: lemon juice 2 tablespoons, parsley 0.25 chopped, and cherry tomatoes 0.25 cup.

Directions:

1. Prepare a medium sized baking sheet by lining with foil

2. Scrub sweet potatoes and cut them into halves.

3. In a large dish, combine the spices and toss the chickpeas into the mixture. Transfer the chickpeas to the sheet.

4. Apply olive oil to the sweet potatoes and place on the sheet. Wait for up to 18 minutes for these two ingredients to roast.

5. Meanwhile, mix all the sauce ingredients in a dish. Stir to combine while adding some water. Season by adding garlic and salt to your liking. Add lemon juice.

6. In a separate dish, toss the tomato and lemon juice

7. Remove the dish from the oven once 18 minutes are over.

8. Switch sides of potatoes and top with the previously made mixtures.

9. Serve while hot.

Dinner: Potatoes with Tuna and Romaine

This is a good meal for dinner, and it is packed with anti-inflammatory properties, especially omega-3 fatty acids. Also, it is a recipe that is easy and quick to prepare.

Total prep & cook time: 30 minutes

Serving yields: 4

Nutritional facts: 611 calories/ 25g net carbs/ 40g total fats/ 39g protein

Ingredients needed: olive oil 0.25 cup, lemon juice 5 drops, black pepper and salt a pinch each, golden potatoes 1 pound and chopped, tuna fillets 6 ounces, melted butter 1 tablespoon, paprika 0.25 teaspoon, and romaine lettuce 2 hearts.

Directions:

1. Prepare a baking sheet.
2. Dip potatoes in olive oil and transfer to the baking sheet.

3. Roast potatoes for 15 minutes at 400 degrees Fahrenheit.

4. Meanwhile, divide the 2 romaine hearts by half and apply olive oil and lemon juice. Add a pinch of salt and black pepper to season. Set aside

5. Spread the tuna fillets with butter. Add paprika, salt and pepper to season.

6. Arrange the fillets and romaine hearts on the baking sheet with the potatoes.

7. Continue to roast contents for up to 5 minutes allowing the tuna and lettuce to cook. Serve while hot.

Breakfast: Warming Carrot Soup

Warming carrot soup is an effective purifier that is anti-inflammatory and help to prevent arthritis and rheumatism. The soup is packed with turmeric and ginger, which makes for a delicious anti-inflammatory meal.

Total prep & cook time: 30 minutes

Serving yields: 4

Nutritional facts: 117 calories/ 5.6g net carbs/ 7g total fats/ 1.2g protein

Ingredients needed: white onion 1, carrots 3, ginger 1-inch ground, garlic cloves 3 ground, vegetable stock 4 cups, turmeric 1-inch ground, coconut milk 0.25 cup, lemon juice 1 tablespoon, white and black sesame seeds, and olive oil 1 tablespoon.

Directions:

1. Put small sized onions and carrots into a medium sized dish.
2. Warm oil in a large cooking pan before adding the turmeric, ginger and garlic. Heat for a minute.
3. Add carrots and vegetables to the pan and reduce heat.Cook for 18 minutes allowing the carrot to cook.
4. Transfer to a blender and mix to achieve a smooth soup.
5. Add in lemon juice. Serve with sesame seeds and coconut milk.

Total prep & cook time: 20   minutes

Serving yields: 4

Nutritional facts: 189 calories/ 0.8g net carbs/ 5.3g total fats/ 0.7g protein

Ingredients needed: peeled shrimp 1.5 pounds, bell peppers 3 sliced, red onion 1 small, olive oil 0.25 cup, salt 0.5 tablespoon, ground pepper 1 tablespoon, chili 1 tablespoon, 0.5 teaspoon each ground cumin, smoked paprika, onion and garlic powder, lime, cilantro and warm tortillas.

Directions:

1. Prepare a baking sheet with tin foil and coat with cooking spray
2. Mix onion, pepper, olive oil, salt and other spices.
3. Place shrimp, onions and bell peppers on the sheet.
4. Cook for 8 minutes at a heat of 450 degrees Fahrenheit.
5. Flip over and cook for 2 more minutes so that the shrimp cooks through.

6. Sprinkle juice from fresh lime and top with cilantro.

7. Put on warm tortillas and serve.

Dinner: Black olives, Kale, and Fennel

This is a delicious Mediterranean-inspired dish. It is easy to prepare and good for dinner. Most importantly, it is packed with anti-inflammatory properties, especially antioxidants.

Total prep & cook time: 30 minutes

Serving yields: 4

Nutritional facts: 257 calories/ 12g net carbs/ 13g total fats/ 23g protein

Ingredients needed: red pepper 1, water 0.5 cup, oregano 1 tablespoon, black olives 1 cup, salt 1 teaspoon, fennel seeds 0.25 tablespoon, Orange zest 1 teaspoon, a pinch of black pepper, chopped kale 2 cups, cut tomatoes 114 ounces, chopped garlic 3 cloves , fennel 2 cups sliced, onion 1 sliced, oregano and olive oil 2 tablespoons.

Directions:

1. Using a large cooking pot, heat the oil and other seasoning elements for 6 minutes.
2. Add fresh tomato, water and kale, and leave to cook for about 6 minutes. Add oregano, olives and red pepper to the mixture and keep cook.
3. Add in fish, pepper, salt, orange zest and fennel seeds. Cover and leave to simmer for 8 minutes.
4. Once out of the oven, sprinkle with more zest, oregano and olive oil. Serve hot.

Breakfast: Strawberry Veggie Smoothie

As discussed, veggies are great for reducing inflammation. The advantage with veggies is that they have significant nutritional value compared to other foods with a larger percentage of calories. In this case, you can choose to use cauliflower or zucchini as the main veggie. When using veggies you can either freeze or steam, whichever you deem appropriate.

Total prep & cook time: 10 minutes

Serving yields: 2

Nutritional facts: 50 calories/ 8g net carbs/ 0.3g total fats/ 0.7g protein

Ingredients needed: vanilla almond milk unsweetened, nut butter 1 tablespoon, strawberries 2 cups frozen or fresh, ice, scoop protein powder, cauliflower 1 cup, and zucchini 1 large.

Directions:

1. Blend a mixture of all ingredients at a high speed
2. Serve and enjoy

Lunch: Paleo Shrimp and Grits

Shrimp is rich in astaxanthin, which is a great antioxidant. Grits are a cruciferous vegetable that helps in suppressing inflammatory responses. This meal is a certainly a satisfying quick fix.

Total prep & cook time: 12 minutes

Serving yields: 2

Nutritional facts: 510 calories/ 3g net carbs/ 33g total fats/ 47g protein

Ingredients needed: Shrimp, a pinch of salt, butter 2 tablespoons, Cajun spice 2 tablespoons, and water 0.5 cup.

For Grits: cauliflower 1 bag 12-ounce, clove garlic 1 large, butter 2 tablespoons, a pinch of salt.

Directions:

1. Boil 0.5 cup water using a medium frying pan
2. Steam cauliflower in a steaming basket and top with garlic. Cover and steam until soft.
3. Put the cauliflower in a food processor and add butter. Add a pinch of salt and the steaming water. Process all ingredients again to ensure smoothness.
4. Prepare shrimp by coating it with cajun seasoning. Set aside.
5. Heat butter in a cooking pan. Add shrimp and cook for about 2 minutes. Flip sides to allow shrimp to cook evenly. It is ready if both sides have turned pink.

6. Remove from heat. Serve while hot.

Total prep & cook time: 20 minutes

Serving yields: 8

Nutritional facts: 305 calories/ 14.5g net carbs/ 26.1g total fats/ 7.5g protein

Ingredients needed: firm tofu 12 ounces, olive oil 1 teaspoon, a pinch of salt, sweet potatoes 2 scrubbed and chopped, green curry paste 4 tablespoons, coconut milk 3 14 ounce cans, and broccoli florets 3 cups.

Directions:

1. Drain the tofu with a sieve. Cut the tofu into small sizes.
2. Heat olive oil and water in a cooking pan.
3. Add tofu and salt, and leave for 10 minutes. Tofu is ready when golden brown.
4. Add coconut milk, sweet potatoes and curry paste to the cooking pot.

5. Simmer for 5 minutes until sweet potatoes become tender. Continue to simmer for 4 minutes to allow the broccoli to cook.
6. Serve while hot.

Additional tip: Can be served with brown rice if preferred

Breakfast: Celery Juice

Celery juice is among the popular trends in the health and healing realm of knowledge. It is a fresh, nourishing, and delicious drink that is easy to make. It reverses inflammation by starving the pathogens that contribute to inflammation. Typically, celery juice is made from the celery plant, a marshland plant that is cultivated as a vegetable.

Total prep & cook time: 15 minutes

Serving yields: 4

Nutritional facts: 40 calories/ 9g net carbs/ 0g total fats/ 2g protein

Ingredients needed: 1 bunch of organic celery and 1 glass of water

Directions:

1. Rinse the celery thoroughly to get rid of dirt
2. Chop the celery into small pieces
3. Run the celery through a blender at a high speed and blend until smooth
4. Strain and drink immediately
5. It is preferably drunk on an empty stomach for effective action
6. Keep increasing the amount of celery relative to water as you get used to the drink, since it is preferably consumed on its own.

Lunch: Rice with Salmon Parcels and Broccoli

This meal is quick to fix up and we already know that yummy salmon and brown rice are some of the best anti-inflammatory foods available.

Total prep & cook time: 30 minutes

Serving yields: 2

Nutritional facts: 561 calories/ 40.5g net carbs/ 5.5g total fats/ 41.1g protein

Ingredients needed: olives cut into pieces 20 grams, cooked brown rice 1 cup, pesto 0.25 cup, lemon 1 chopped, salmon fillets 5, and broccoli 1 cup.

Directions:

1. Prepare a baking sheet by spraying with cooking spray.
2. Add the rice and olives to a bowl and stir to combine.
3. Add pesto, basil and lemon juice and mix thoroughly. Place on baking sheet.
4. Place fish fillets on top of the mixture on the baking sheet. Add any residual pesto, the broccoli and lemon slices on top.
5. Cover the mixture with foil, covering all sides.
6. Put the package on a baking pan and let it cook for 23 minutes.
7. Remove from heat and serve while hot.

Dinner: Garlic Paleo Whole Noodles

This is one of the easiest and quickest meals to make, packed with antioxidants and fiber.

Total prep & cook time: 10 minutes

Serving yields: 4

Nutritional facts: 389 calories/ 62g net carbs/ 15g total fats/ 6g protein

Ingredients needed: cooked spaghetti squash 1, zucchini and carrot 1 small each, bell pepper 1, cilantro 0.5 cup, peanuts 0.25 cup roasted.

For the sauce: medjool dates 6, garlic cloves 4, fish sauce 0.25 cup, red curry paste 4 teaspoons, ground ginger 4 teaspoons, coconut milk 0.25 cup, coconut aminos 0.5 cup.

Directions:

1. Blend all sauce ingredients until smooth.
2. Mix noodle ingredients in a dish and let them combine thoroughly.Add to pan and heat.
3. Add sauce to pan and allow to warm.

4. Serve hot.

Breakfast: Scrambled Eggs with Turmeric

It is important to note that eggs contain a large amount of protein. Egg yolk are notable for containing vitamin D which is capable of hindering the body's inflammation process because it positively impacts the immune system. Also, turmeric provides an anti-inflammatory boost when used with scrambled eggs.

Turmeric contains a significant amount of curcumin which helps manage inflammatory and oxidative conditions. Most people eat breakfast after exercising, and eggs are suitable at such times because they boost recovery post exercise due to their high potassium and protein content. In this case, it is good to use spinach because it helps in nourishing the digestive system and supporting detoxification.

Total prep & cook time: 20 minutes

Serving yields: 2

Nutritional facts: calories 155/ net carbs 1.1 g/ total fats 11 g/ protein 14 g

Ingredients needed: organic or free-range eggs 4, fresh grated turmeric 1 teaspoon, cream or organic coconut milk 1 teaspoon, super greens pesto 1 tablespoon, baby spinach leaves 100g, cold pressed olive oil 2 teaspoons and pinch sea salt.

Directions:

1. In a mixing bowl add together the eggs, sea salt, coconut milk, chia and turmeric and combine to make a good mixture.
2. Into a cooking pan, pour 1 teaspoon of olive oil and heat, then add the pesto and spinach cooking for half a minute until the spinach leaves are wilted. Remove from heat.
3. Put 1 teaspoon of olive oil in a non-stick cooking pan and heat.
4. Empty into the pan, the egg mixture
5. Gently stir the mixture until the eggs begin to set and get creamy. Add the spinach.
6. Serve and enjoy.

Lunch: Hazelnut, Beetroot, and Lentil Salad

This is a good lunch especially if you are a vegetarian or on a vegetarian diet. Lentil salad is simple to prepare and is rich in proteins. Hazelnuts contain vitamin E and provide protein, while beetroot and lentils increase fiber content. Vitamin E is accredited as an excellent antioxidant. Additionally, beetroots provide a significant amount of betaine which is antioxidant and anti-inflammatory. This lunch will be completed with a warm ginger dressing.

Total prep & cook time: 15 minutes

Serving yields: 3

Nutritional facts: calories 670 / net carbs 20 g / total fats 60g / protein 30g

Ingredients needed: Sea salt, cooked beetroot 3 chopped into small pieces, lentils 1 cup, filtered water 2 ¾ cup, onions 2 large well sliced, chopped hazelnuts 2 tablespoons, a fresh mint that is unevenly sliced and roughly cut fresh parsley.

For the ginger dressing: fresh ginger ¾ inch cube peeled and sliced, olive oil 6 tablespoons, dijon mustard 1 tablespoon, apple cider vinegar 2 teaspoons, salt a pinch and black pepper each.

Directions:

1. Place lentils in a cooking pan and add the water. Bring the mixture to a boil and then simmer for 14 minutes until the water has evaporated and you are left with cooked lentils. Remove the lentil from the cooking pan for cooling.
2. After the lentils have cooled add onions, herbs, hazelnuts, beetroot, and mix to thoroughly combine.
3. Combine vinegar, oil, mustard, and ginger and blend until everything is mixed.
4. Add the dressing to the salad and serve.

Dinner: Vegetable Curry and Shrimp

Shrimp contains astaxanthin, an anti-inflammatory and antioxidant. In addition, the peas, red peppers, carrots are great because they contain healthful polyphenol. The advantage with turmeric is that it is somehow tasteless and can be used in any casserole, soups, or curry. It is convenient to prepare and you will only need a few ingredients. If you do not like curry you can use basil, pepper, salt, or garlic instead.

Total prep & cook time: 30 minutes

Serving yields: 4

Nutritional facts: calories 170 / net carbs 2 g / Total fats 7 g/ Protein 7 g

Ingredients needed: coconut oil or butter 3 tablespoons, curry powder 3 tablespoons, onion 1 sliced, coconut milk 1 cup, cauliflower 1 head, and shrimp, tails removed.

Directions:

1. Place coconut oil in a pan and heat. Add the sliced onion.
2. Fry onions until they are slightly soft.
3. Steam the vegetables.
4. Add curry seasoning and coconut milk.
5. Cook for a few minutes to integrate flavors.

6. Add thawed shrimp and cook for at least seven minutes until the shrimp are well cooked.
7. Serve with steamed veggies.

Breakfast: Poached Eggs, Avocado, & Smoked Salmon on Toast

Don't be surprised by this combination, it is one of the best-known anti-inflammatory fact that avocado and salmon contain a high amount of omega-3 fatty acids. It has been proven that healthful fatty acids can help improve a person's heart health. It helps in lowering the risk of cardiovascular disease. Moreover, this breakfast is suitable especially during active days because it comes together so fast.

Total prep & cook time: 30 minutes

Serving yields: 1

Nutritional facts: calories 200/ net carbs 1g / total fats 12g/ protein 25g

Ingredients needed: Freshly squeezed lemon juice ¼ tablespoon, smashed avocado, toasted bread 2 slices, scallions 1 tablespoon thinly sliced, a splash of Kikkoman soy sauce, eggs 2, smoked salmon 3.5 oz., and a pinch of cracked black pepper and salt.

Directions:

1. In a small dish, smash the avocado.
2. Add salt and lemon juice. Mix ingredients thoroughly.
3. Toast the bread and poach two eggs.
4. On both sides of the toasted bread spread the avocado and then place salmon on both sides.
5. Place a poached egg on each slice.
6. You can apply pepper or soy sauce and accompany this with micro greens and scallions.

Lunch: Beans with Cauliflower Steak and Tomatoes

This meal is a suitable alternative to steak, especially for vegetarians. Cauliflower contains a significantly high antioxidant and fiber source. Women who eat more cruciferous vegetables tend to have lower inflammation.

Total prep & cook time: 30 minutes

Serving yields: 2

Nutritional facts: calories 400/ net carbs 70g / total fats 2.4g / protein 30g

Ingredients needed: cauliflower 1 head large, oil 0.5 cup, salt, black pepper 1 teaspoon, trimmed green beans, finely cut garlic cloves 3, lemon zest 0.75 teaspoons finely grated, parsley 1/3 teaspoon, panko 1/3 cup. white beans 1 can, parmesan 0.25 cup well grated, red cherry tomatoes 1 can, mayonnaise 3 tablespoons, and dijon mustard 1 teaspoon.

Directions:

1. Heat the oven at 425-degrees Fahrenheit.Toss green beans with a ½ teaspoon salt, 1 tablespoon oil and pepper on a rimmed baking sheet.Roast them until they begin to blister.
2. Prepare the cauliflower by placing it head side down and making a cut in its center to make two steaks. Brush both sides of the cauliflower with 1 tablespoon of oil placed. Season it with pepper or salt. Roast it, waiting for the cauliflower to turn brown and tender.

3. Take a medium-sized bowl, whisking garlic, ½ tablespoon pepper, 1 ¼ teaspoon salt, and ½ teaspoon pepper.Add parmesan and panko

4. In a second bowl mix the tomatoes and beans.

5. Remove baking sheet from over and spread mayonnaise over cauliflower. Spread panko mixture equally over cauliflower. Combine the beans on the sheet. Then put them back to the oven for a few minutes.

6. Then serve the white beans, green beans, cauliflower and tomatoes.

Dinner: Slow Cooker Turkey Chili

A big bowl of chili provides nutrients and warmth. Foods that are high in salt are suitable for promoting fluid retention. For low salt use fresh jalapenos or choosing low-sodium canned beans. It is a delicious meal itself but you can use a little organic non-fat fresh avocado and Greek yogurt. The following recipe is healthy and easy to make.

Total prep & cook time: 15 minutes

Serving yields: 6

Nutritional facts: calories 189 / net carbs 0.1g / total fats 7 g/ protein 29g

Ingredients needed: olive oil, pre-cooked turkey, diced onion 1, cut red pepper, sliced yellow pepper 1, deli-sliced tamed jalapeno peppers 1 jar, beans red 2 cups, beans black 2 cups, petite cut tomatoes, tomato sauce, salt and black pepper, cumin 1 tablespoon, chili powder 2 tablespoons and frozen corn 1 cup. Also, you may have Greek yogurt, shredded cheese, and green onions for topping options.

Directions:

1. Cook the turkey in the skillet until it turns brown.
2. Transfer turkey into the slow cooker.
3. Add the chili powder, onions, corn, jalapenos, beans, tomato sauce, diced tomatoes, peppers, and cumin.
4. Heat on high for 7 hours
5. Season to your liking
6. Serve while hot

Granola with pumpkin and sunflower seeds is one of the healthiest breakfasts. You can use it together with soy yogurt and almond milk which would make for an energizing breakfast. It is easy to make snacks with granola too.

Total prep & cook time: 20 minutes

Serving yields: 3

Nutritional facts: calories 340 / net carbs 75g / Total fats 2g / Protein 11g

Ingredients needed: ginger, oats 2 cups, buckwheat 1 cup, pitted dates 1.5 cups, apple puree/sauce 1 cup, sunflower seeds 1 cup, coconut oil 6 tablespoons, cocoa powder 4 tablespoons.

Directions:

1. Preheat the oven to 180 degrees Celsius.
2. Mix together the seeds, oats, and buckwheat in a dish

3. Add coconut oil, apple puree and dates into a sauce pan and simmer for 5 minutes until the dates become soft.
4. When the dates are soft place them into a blender and add the cocoa powder.
5. After blending, add the mix to the seed, oat and buckwheat mixture, stirring completely until everything is covered.
6. Heat a large frying pan with coconut oil, add the mixture and then place it in the oven to bake.
7. Once it is crispy, remove and allow it to cool, storing in an airtight container for up to 30 days or more.

Lunch: Sweet Potato Soup and Roasted Red Pepper

This is a superb, antioxidant-rich soup. You can prepare it a week early during your free time and store it because it freezes so easily. It is important that you roast the sweet potatoes early enough. Roasted red peppers are suitable to reduce the sodium here.

Total prep & cook time: 30 minutes

Serving yields: 3

Nutritional facts: calories 86/ net carbs 20g / Total fats 0.1g / protein 1.6g

Ingredients needed: minced fresh cilantro 0.25 cup, olive oil 0.25 cup, ground coriander 1 teaspoon, onion 1 chopped, roasted red peppers 1 jar, diced green chills 4 ounce, vegetable broth 4 cups, ground cumin 1 tablespoon, salt 1 teaspoon, peeled and cubed sweet potatoes 4 cups, cream cheese cubed 4 oz. and lemon juice 2 teaspoons.

Directions:

1. Heat the oil in a large soup dish then add the chopped onion and cook until softened. Add in the green chills, coriander, salt, red peppers, and cumin. Cook for 1 to 2 minutes.
2. Mix juice from roasted red peppers, vegetable broth, sweet potatoes and bring to a boil. Simmer until the potatoes become tender, approximately 15 minutes.
3. Mix in the lemon juice and cilantro and then leave it to cool.

4. Blend some of the soup together with the cream cheese. When it becomes smooth, add it back into the soup dish and heat.
5. If you need to, you can season with additional salt.

Dinner: Broiled Salmon with Spinach

Both fish and veggies are good inflammation fighting ingredient and to prepare this meal you do not require any fancy cooking skills. It is a combination of two superfoods, forming a flavorful meal that you can prepare in 20 minutes.

Total prep & cook time: 20 minutes

Serving yields: 1

Nutritional facts: calories 154/ net carbs 10g/ Total fats 9.8g / Protein 2g

Ingredients needed: fresh wild salmon 4 oz., Dijon mustard 1.5 tablespoons, low sodium soy sauce 0.25 cup, steamed spinach 1 cup and salt to taste

Directions:

1. Start by heating a cooking pan over medium heat
2. Spread mustard over the surface of the salmon and sprinkle soy sauce on its top.
3. Place the salmon in the pan and cook for ten minutes or until it is thoroughly cooked.Steam the spinach while waiting for salmon to cook

Top salmon with spinach then add pepper or salt for taste.

Conclusion

Inflammation is a serious health issue. There are two main conditions of inflammation: acute and chronic inflammation. In most cases, people experience acute inflammation, and it is characterized simply by pain. While inflammation is suitable for the healing process of an infection or an injury, when the body releases excessive white blood cells where there is no infection or injury, a situation where healthy cells are attacked ensues.

Acute inflammation, in this sense, is for the most part beneficial, but it is also associated with unpleasant symptoms such as itching, sore throat, and other pains. It is paramount to note that there are various factors that stimulate inflammation and which include tissue death, unsuitable immunological responses, chemicals, physical agents and microorganisms. Their approach in causing inflammation varies according to many factors. (For instance, endotoxins which initiate inflammation through radiation, burns and physical trauma.) Chronic inflammation is a more serious situation and is shown in conjunction with serious diseases such as lung disease, heart disease, and rheumatoid arthritis.

Despite being a scary condition, inflammation can actually be satisfactorily addressed in many situations through anti-inflammatory diets. In the above case of 14 days, recipes have been discussed which are only a sample of the numerous meals that a person can try. These are diets that are rich in nutrients and helpful to the body compared to sugary foods that have become the order of the day among most people. As shown, the diet requires a maximum of 30 minutes or less to prepare with some having the advantage of storing to the freezer so you can use in a few days. Most people claim that cooking is time-consuming and expensive and that they would rather eat take away, fries, chicken among other forms of junk foods. However, compromising your health is more expensive and it far more worthwhile to be cautious of what you consume.

Some of the discussed aspects or rather, tips, in relation to anti-inflammatory diets include the following: Eating a variety of vegetables and fruits has proven to be significantly helpful as well as ensuring that you avoid or eat only a little amount of fast food. Eliminating sugary beverages such as soda is helpful. It will be helpful to be make plans for food shopping to ensure that you are well planned to gather healthful snacks and meals. Drinking water and meeting daily calorie requirements and exercising regularly is also essential. Supplements such as turmeric and omega-3 are important to your diet and ensuring that you are getting an adequate amount of sleep is absolutely necessary.

It has been discussed that inflammation is a bodily response to illnesses, including injury or infection. In this condition, the body releases many white blood cells in the area where there is an injury or infection. Inflammation is worse when it reaches chronic levels and results in such diseases as asthma, psoriasis, and arthritis. In such situations the immune system goes into overdrive and attacks healthy tissues.

Inflammation can be reduced by taking various prescribed medications. However, a suitable way to address it is through an anti-inflammatory diet. As noted, the issue of diet is confusing to most people as a large percentage of what is consumed on a daily basis makes one more susceptible to inflammation. Through an anti-inflammatory diet, a person is able to reduce the inflammatory body response.

An anti-inflammatory diet is characterized by nutrients instead of sugary foods. Also, it contains antioxidants which protect the body against the risk of certain diseases. For instance, whole grain and fish are identified as good foods, reducing the effects of inflammation on the cardiovascular system.

This book has explained that anti-inflammatory diets are suitable for addressing heart disease, obesity, diabetes, colitis, and rheumatoid arthritis. The foods to avoid include excess alcohol, white pasta, white bread, gluten, sugary drinks and processed meats, among others. Important anti-inflammatory foods include olives, avocados, green tea, beans and lentils, dark red berries and blueberries, among others. The most essential aspects noted here is that having a well-planned diet that would play a vital role in addressing inflammation.

Thank you for making it through to the end of The Anti-

Inflammatory Diet, let's hope it was enjoyable and informative and has provided you with all of the tools you need to achieve your goals whatever they may be.

The next step is to put this new information to action. Go to the grocery store and fill that cart with colorful, anti-inflammatory foods and start your new healthy, pain free life .

Finally, if you found this book has changed your life or is useful in any way, a review on Amazon is always appreciated!

Mely Johnson

Made in the USA
San Bernardino, CA
06 February 2020

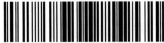